If you are ever in a ho
possibly grief—and yo
Especially if you are tr
chair and knows your
comfort and healing to
Scripture, prayers, pro

suffering—is a great res ....t draining away. No
God talk, just talk about the faithfulness of God and how to embrace it.
DANIEL TAYLOR PHD
AUTHOR, *CREATING A SPIRITUAL LEGACY, DEATH COMES FOR THE DECONSTRUCTIONIST* (A NOVEL)

With acute accuracy Elizabeth names my deepest fears;
With gentle probing she invites me to trust my Father;
With an economy of words she creates space for faith to flourish.
SHARI THOMAS
FOUNDER AND EXECUTIVE DIRECTOR OF PARAKALEO

This brilliant book is a tender gift of the presence of God for those caught in the
deep woods of medical uncertainty. When we are in the hospital waiting for resolution, we don't need a long chapter of admonitions or vague mumblings of comfort.
We need a guide who has traversed this terrain and has a compass and a map to help
us orient our journey. Elizabeth Turnage offers a wisdom that has been hard won,
meets the test of the gospel, and is beautifully and brilliantly written. I can't recommend this book more highly than to say you need a copy for yourself and eventually
for every friend or family member who is called to wait for redemption.
DAN B. ALLENDER PHD
PROFESSOR OF COUNSELING PSYCHOLOGY
FOUNDING PRESIDENT, THE SEATTLE SCHOOL OF THEOLOGY AND PSYCHOLOGY

Elizabeth writes to anyone who finds themselves in the waiting room of God's sover-
eign purposes. She meets us there as an empathetic friend reminding us what is true
in His Word, urging us to listen to the refreshing lyrics of the gospel. She beautifully
models what it means to lift our eyes to the Father who is faithful to meet us in the
midst of our suffering.
KAREN HODGE
COORDINATOR OF WOMEN'S MINISTRIES
PRESBYTERIAN CHURCH IN AMERICA (PCA)

Waiting is a part of life. We wait in lines, to hear from a college, to get a job, to
find a spouse, to have a baby, for a wayward child to return…. And we wait in
medical waiting rooms: for a diagnosis, through a surgery, for news—hopefully
good, too often bad. Elizabeth Turnage, in *The Waiting Room*, sits with us, offering

understanding, peace and courage. She takes us right to our God through her personal story of waiting room ordeals, through God's Word, in prayer. And she conveys perspective for the difficulty of today, comfort and strength for the ongoing journey and great hope for the future. This is a helpful book for all the waiting of our lives.

JUDY DOUGLASS
WRITER, SPEAKER, ENCOURAGER
DIRECTOR, CRU WOMEN'S RESOURCES

The Waiting Room records naked, raw truth about "The Club" of those who have suffered deep loss. Elizabeth's honesty about her family trauma will draw you in and challenge your core assumptions. She invites you to refocus on the hope that disease, tears, and death are on a short leash. She invites you to engage scripture, worship music, prayer, and honesty with your Creator. This is a book that I will read multiple times as Elizabeth has shown me where God is in plain sight in the wilderness of suffering.

DR. PENNY NELSON FREEMAN
LICENSED COUNSELOR AND TRAINER

The Waiting Room will comfort me when I take a loved one to the hospital. Elizabeth's love for Jesus and Scripture helps us when life is on pause. Her words guide us along green pastures and still waters when the noise from our fear seems overwhelming. I strongly recommend her book to anyone that has to wait as a dear one suffers.

REBECCA ALLENDER
CO-FOUNDER, THE ALLENDER CENTER; AUTHOR, *HIDDEN IN PLAIN SIGHT*

Elizabeth Turnage has often penned gracious and wise words that lead us back to gospel truth. In this interactive meditation, Elizabeth shares her own personal walk through pain and suffering. She writes with amazing clarity and honesty and makes the dark, painful moments as real to the reader as they were to her. While you journey with her through these hard spaces, you will also see how she found the light of God's mercy and grace shining in the dark. Your heart will resonate with the struggle and be encouraged by the scriptures and prayer points. If you allow yourself to take this interactive journey of meditation, you may well find a place where your own heart will grow in trust and grace, even in the hard.

RUTH ANN BATSTONE
COUNSELOR AND MENTOR, SERGE; SENIOR STAFF CONSULTANT, PARAKALEO

Dear Becky —
Your compassionate
concern and your fierce
and fervent prayer.

THE

WAITING

ROOM

60 MEDITATIONS FOR FINDING
PEACE & HOPE IN A HEALTH CRISIS

carried me from afar
during a terrifying season.
I am so grateful to
have you in my corner!
Love, Elizabeth

Elizabeth Reynolds Turnage

FOREWORD BY SCOTTY SMITH

Living Story
www.elizabethturnage.com
etlivingstory@gmail.com

Volume discounts are available. Please contact the publisher at etlivingstory@gmail.com for information.
Cover and interior design: Erik M. Peterson.
Page composition: Charity Walton with Good Shepherd Publications

ISBN: 978-0-9980321-0-8 (print)
ISBN: 978-0-9980321-1-5 (ebook)
Library of Congress Control Number: 2018913459

Names: Turnage, Elizabeth Reynolds, author. | Smith, Scotty, 1950-, foreword author.

Title: The Waiting room : 60 meditations for finding peace and hope in a health crisis / Elizabeth Reynolds Turnage ; foreword by Scotty Smith.

Description: Includes bibliographical references and index. | Pensacola, FL: Living Story, 2019.

Identifiers: LCCN 2018913459 | ISBN 9780998032108 (pbk.) | 9780998032115 (ebook)

Subjects: LCSH Health--Religious aspects | Caregivers--Prayers and devotions. | Sick--Prayers and devotions. | Consolation. | Cancer--Patients--Prayers and devotions. | Christian literature--Prayers. | Anxiety--Religious aspects--Christianity. | Peace of mind--Religious aspects--Christianity. | BISAC RELIGION / Christian Living / Devotional | BODY, MIND & SPIRIT / Healing / Prayer & Spiritual

Classification: LCC BV4910 .T87 2019 | DDC 242/.4--dc23

Table of Contents

Foreword. ix
The Back Story xiii
Introduction xvii
How This Book Is Designed xxi
Your Only Comfort. 1
You Are Forgiven. 3
Becoming Mature and Complete 7
God Rules Everything. 11
Don't Panic—He's Got You. 15
How to Pray 19
Knowledge That Will Change Your World 23
God Knows You 27
Live by Every Word. 31
Your Troubled Heart 35
Sharing the Story 39
Prayer Requests: Inviting Community to Pray. 43
Looking for a Better Place. 47
Our Ultimate Question. 51
God's Answer 55
Comfort as You Have Been Comforted. 59
I Know Whom I Have Believed 63
Loss of Dignity 67
Normal Grief 71
Change of Plans 75
'Tis So Sweet to Trust in Jesus 79
When You Are Lonely. 83
Your Helper is Here! 87
Unfulfilled 91
All Will Be Well 95
Patience and Patients. 99
Never Give Up 103
My Peace I Give 107
The Peace of God 111

The Community of Faith 115

When You Are Weak........................ 119

Self-Care: Your Body Is a Temple 123

Searching for Signs of Redemption 127

When God Said "No" 131

When You Mistake Jesus for a Ghost. 135

Steadfast 139

Jesus Has His Eyes on You. 143

The Kindness of Strangers 147

The Embrace of the Father 151

The Wrong Question........................ 155

Jesus Wept. 159

Worth Waiting For 163

The Gentleness of Jesus...................... 167

The Lord Is Near........................... 171

Mat-Friends 175

What Is Healing? 179

Termites, Tumors, and Other Hidden Dangers 183

Count Your Losses 187

Count Your Blessings 191

Nothing Can Separate Us 195

Return to Normal 199

A Good Scar Story 203

Grieving in Uncertainty 207

Do You Believe in Miracles? 211

Everyday Miracles.......................... 215

An Angelic Army 219

Tough Decisions........................... 223

The First Enemy: Satan 227

The Final Enemy: Death...................... 231

The Wait Is Over! 235

Acknowledgments.......................... 239

Appendix 241

Notes 245

Scripture Index 249

Complete Song List......................... 253

Foreword

THANKFUL FOR FIVE green lights out of six, I pushed, then broke the posted speed limit, as I raced to the nearest walk-in clinic. As Darlene struggled for her next breath, my rational concerns gave way to escalating fears. "What if we don't make it in time? How do you do CPR when someone's having an asthma attack? How long will we have to wait in medical-lobby-purgatory?"

This story isn't from years ago, but days ago. Fortunately, we did make it to the Vanderbilt Walk-in Clinic in time and were greeted by an empty waiting room, as well as a nurse who rushed Darlene into a room for a breathing treatment. Soon, a most compassionate doctor provided great care and we were on our way home in less than an hour.

But that's not always the case, right? All of us have stories of being stuck between the weight of uncertainty and the wait for good medical care—and the wait—hopefully, for healing.

Whether it's an hour in the office lobby of a trusted, family doctor; or the long hours (days, weeks) spent at home waiting for pathology reports, medical treatments, or therapy results; or those unexpected health emergencies that happen on family vacations, out-of-town celebrations, or out-of-country missions trips—waiting is frustrating, inconvenient, and fear-fueling—a veritable incubator for vulnerability.

That's why I am so excited about Elizabeth Turnage's new book, *The Waiting Room*. My friend writes with a heart bent on bringing peace and hope into the fear-full space of health crises. She writes as someone who walks closely with the God of all mercy and grace. She writes as trained story-coach, gospel-discipler, and life-counselor. But she also writes as someone who has learned to steward her own health struggles, and the stories of those she loves.

During our treasured fifteen-year friendship with Elizabeth and Kip Turnage, we two couples have buried parents after long illnesses and walked with friends through all kinds of health difficulties. We've also experienced many of our own medical challenges. Between Elizabeth and me, I think the two of us have tallied about fourteen orthopedic surgeries. Elizabeth has logged many, many hours waiting!

But as you'll soon find out, the most recent impetus for this raw, real, and encouraging collection of meditations, is the health-care journey Elizabeth and Kip have been walking with their son, Robert—their youngest of four children. That's her story to tell, but here's my encouragement to offer.

As a pastor for the past four decades, I have longed for a book just like this one—for my own benefit, but also to put into the hands of women and men like yourself. Whether you are currently in the "waiting room" for yourself, or with someone you love—no matter your faith story—past or present, open your heart and this little book. Elizabeth offers real hope, not pious hype; a validation of our pain, not sentimental spin; the journey towards lasting peace, not a recipe for temporary relief.

It hasn't escaped my attention that I am writing this foreword during Advent in 2018. In the Christian calendar, Advent is a season of waiting with hope for Christmas Day—the celebration and implications of Jesus' birth. It is my prayer, as you read Elizabeth's sixty brief chapters, that you will come to understand the gospel of God's grace—the good news of Jesus Christ, in fresh and palpable ways.

This is the life-giving aroma that permeates every page of this book. This is the gentleness and kindness that met Elizabeth, time after time, in her waiting room. This is the peace and hope that is offered to each one of us.

SCOTTY SMITH — PASTOR EMERITUS CHRIST COMMUNITY CHURCH, FRANKLIN, TN
TEACHER IN RESIDENCE, WEST END COMMUNITY CHURCH, NASHVILLE, TN

The Back Story

IT WAS THE SUMMER of 2017, and it seemed that the waiting room had become my new home. The sturdy chairs, the durable flooring, the unflattering light—I had a lot of time to observe the details. I had been thrust into that season in the waiting room—both as a caregiver of loved ones and a mourner of lost ones—and then left with a great deal of time for reflection. And while I waited, seemingly forever, I began to wonder how God might be working in that wilderness of waiting.

In June and July, my eighty-three-year-old Dad, who had been diagnosed with Stage IV prostate cancer two years before, had new metastases in his hips. My mom underwent knee replacement surgery in Atlanta and then had a second surgery for a complication. I was the primary caregiver to both of them during their health crises.

Further health crises and loss hit in late July and August. Our daughter-in-law's beloved grandmother passed away from the effects of lung cancer. My precious uncle had a severe stroke. On August 1, my husband's father had a mild heart attack, then underwent open heart surgery on August 3.

On the same day as my father-in-law's open-heart surgery, our truly excruciating season in the waiting room began. Our twenty-two-year-old son, who was preparing to leave for graduate school in vocal performance, had a sinus Cat scan (CT) to evaluate chronic sinus congestion. The CT revealed a mass on our son's brain. He would need a follow-up MRI. And the waiting began.

Over the next month, our son underwent two separate surgeries to remove the mass in his brain. The first one was stopped when the surgeon believed that what he saw was not a tumor. After further testing, it was decided there was still a tumor, and a second surgery was performed two weeks later. This surgery proved successful—98% of the tumor was removed.

AS SEPTEMBER BEGAN, we continued to wait: for the pathology report, and for our son's recovery. He was doing fairly well, considering the risks of losing motor function after such surgery. He was quiet and rather apathetic, as the doctor had cautioned he might be, but he had only very minor and temporary neurological defects.

Three weeks later, we received the preliminary pathology reports. The tumor was believed to be low grade, but because it had some "interesting and difficult-to-diagnose findings," it had been sent to a world-expert pathologist. We endured more waiting to hear his findings.

That same day, as a resident was removing staples from my son's wound, he discovered discolored fluid, signaling infection. A flurry of activity began, and we were suddenly thrust back into waiting rooms to get labs and another CT scan to determine how deep the infection went.

The next day, the surgeon opened our son's skull for the third time in a matter of five weeks. He washed out the wound and determined that part of the skull was infected, so he removed a small section of bone, then stapled his head back together. Three days later, our son and I left for home. He had a PICC

(Peripherally Inserted Central Catheter) line and a prescription for six weeks of IV antibiotics to be administered by us.

On October 1, we received a call from the neuro-oncologist. The report was back from the California pathologist: the mass was *not cancer*. It was, in fact, a mass of neurons that had probably been in his brain all of his life. We were stunned by the miraculously good news.

We took a moment to breathe deeply. But we quickly discovered that our season in the waiting room had already taken a toll—and further trials were to come.

Our attention had been focused on our son, but his health issues were not the only ones in our lives during that six-week period. My uncle had passed away. My father-in-law had been released from the hospital and entered cardiac rehab. And finally, unbeknownst to me, my father's condition had worsened. Just after our son's third surgery, my dad revealed to me that his oral chemotherapy medications were no longer working, and that he had refused traditional chemotherapy. We were now thrust into the maelstrom of end-of-life decisions in pursuit of relief from the agony he was experiencing. Just two weeks later, on October 11, my dad passed away.

Five days after my dad's death, home health care called to tell us our son's labs indicated he was severely immunosuppressed. Once again, he was sent for further testing—and we were back in the waiting room. The doctors changed his medication, and we once again waited to see if the changes in medicine would reverse the immunosuppression.

Finally, two weeks later, on October 31, the doctors determined that the infection was cured. On December 18, the neuro-oncologist assured us that all diagnostic procedures indicated our son was currently cancer-free and advised following up with him in one year.

In March of 2018, our son underwent his fourth and, we hope, final craniotomy to insert a synthetic plate in his skull to replace the piece of infected bone that had been removed. Following this surgery, he faced several complications but was ultimately declared "healed."

This is the story I was living when I began to look for God in the waiting room.

Introduction

MY EIGHTY-ONE-YEAR-OLD DAD had not been to a doctor in forty years when his health crisis began. On our first visit to the urologist, we walked into a waiting room packed with people—mostly infirm-looking men aged seventy-and-up, along with their caregivers: wives, daughters, sons, and paid workers. My Dad, generally stoic, rarely whiny, took one look at the crowded room and complained, "Oh man, I don't want to be here!"

I shot back, "Oh yeah, Dad, why don't we get a show of hands? Let's ask, 'How many of you are excited to be here—raise your hand!'"

It was a response that seemed aptly worded for me by the Holy Spirit.

Thankfully, my dad saw the humor and burst out laughing. We both gained perspective in that moment. After all, most people don't want to be *here*: in the midst of a health crisis that requires them to visit many doctors and wait in many rooms.

WHAT ABOUT YOU? WHAT IS YOUR EXPERIENCE OF THE WAITING ROOM?

Does your heart pound?

Do your palms sweat?

Does it feel like acid is burning a hole through your chest?

Does your mind race, combing through all of the dreadful possibilities?

WHAT IF...

What if it's cancer?

What if my loved one can never drive again, play tennis again, kiss me again?

What if…my loved one loses her job?

What if…my loved one has six months to live?

Whether you are the caregiver or the patient, the "what-if's" can feel terrifying, and the wait can feel agonizing.

ROOM FOR HOPE

During our son's health crisis, which coincided with the final months of my Dad's life, I sat in many varied waiting rooms. During seemingly endless spells in such spaces, I began to wonder—*what if*—this space could make space for another, better kind of waiting?

- What if…the waiting room could become a *hoping room*, a place to grow our hope?

- What if…in this waiting room, we could discover the surpassing peace of Christ?

- What if…in this waiting room, our eyes could open to the glory and goodness of God?

- What if…in this waiting room, we could discover that as God allows our bodies to be broken, his mercy is working to reconstruct us, to refashion us into people who are more like our suffering Savior, God's Son Jesus?

- What if…in this waiting room, we could see that he is coming to heal not merely all broken brains and hearts and limbs, but more importantly, to heal our deepest wounds caused by our own sins and the sins of others?

Is redemption of the waiting room season possible?

The gospel says it is.

EARTHLY HOPE VS. BIBLICAL HOPE

To understand this redemption, we first need to grasp the difference between earthly hope and biblical hope. Earthly hope focuses on significant, but, in perspective, smaller stories; biblical hope focuses on the crucial and life-transforming Story God is writing in our hearts, in his kingdom, for his glory and our good.

Earthly hope focuses on good outcomes in the here and now or at least the near future. We *hope* that the surgeon can fix our wrecked knee; we *hope* that our son's tumor will be benign; we *hope* that this antibiotic cures the infection. These are all good things to hope for, but we can have no certainty that they will happen.

The Bible teaches that there is a better hope we await: an outcome that is certain and sure. To understand this hope, we need to know the whole story Scripture tells.

THE BIG STORY GOD IS WRITING

In the beginning, God created humans in his image and designed them with a purpose: to glorify and enjoy him (Genesis 1-2). Within a short time, though, humans listened to the evil one, who tempted them to believe that God was holding out on them, that God was not good. They disobeyed their Creator God, taking life into their own hands when they ate the fruit God had forbidden them to eat (Genesis 3).

As a result, sin entered the world (Romans 5:12), and ever since, all humans have been born in sin and have suffered its disastrous effects: death, disease, destruction, and division. But the ever-faithful, always-loving God did not leave us in this miserable condition. He sent his beloved, holy Son into the world to save us from our sins (Isaiah 53:4-5).

In the current season of God's story, those who trust in Christ as Savior know the freedom from guilt and sin that he has brought us (Galatians 5:1). And yet, we still live in a world that is tainted by evil. Drunk drivers have accidents. Political leaders oppress. People pollute rivers and oceans. We harm those we love with our words. Those we love get sick. Those we love die. Every day, we sin; every day we suffer the effects of sin.

All who love Jesus Christ groan alongside all of creation as we await the end of God's Story and its accompanying glory, the final healing of all broken things (Romans 8:18-19):

- In that day, we will be made like him (1 John 3:2).

- In that day, God will wipe away all our tears, and death will be no more (Revelation 21:4).

- In that day, God will dwell with us, and we will never again be separated from the One who completely satisfies our hearts (Revelation 21:3).

- In that day, we will finally live as God designed us, glorifying and enjoying God fully and forever (Isaiah 43:7).

That is what we are really waiting for.

The waiting rooms of a health crisis offer us the surprising opportunity to learn to wait in hope, to make more room in our hearts for the coming of the Lord in all of his glory.

This little book of meditations is intended to help you find peace and hope by drawing your heart to the bigger story God is writing in this small—though profoundly significant—story you are living. May the Word and words, *the* Story and the stories, lead your heart to rest in the One who made you and loves you and waits for you to live with him forever.

How This Book Is Designed

MEDITATIONS FOR PEACE AND HOPE

ALTHOUGH MEDITATION HAS gained popularity in the twenty-first century as a means of achieving calm, God encouraged it long ago. The Bible uses the word *meditate* to refer to the practice of going over the works of God and the Word of God in your mind.[1] The Hebrew word literally means to "chew on," as a cow chews its cud, or as a dog gnaws on a bone. We are to let God's Word marinate in our hearts, captivate our thoughts, and integrate our lives. As we meditate on God's Word, our hearts ease, we fix our hopes on the certain future to come, and we know the peace that surpasses all understanding.

The meditations in these pages are arranged according to some of the varied topics, experiences and emotions you might encounter during this waiting room season.

SCRIPTURE

Each meditation begins with a verse of Scripture. Read it over several times—aloud if you dare—others in the waiting room may need to hear it too! If you have time, read the Scriptures listed at the end of each meditation under "Further Encouragement."

PRAYER

When we are in crisis, it can be hard to know what to pray.

Use the short prayer at the end of each meditation or simply use your own words. You may choose to record these prayers in a separate prayer journal. No matter what approach you take, remember that the Lord loves to hear your voice and to answer your prayers with his Word of hope.

FURTHER ENCOURAGEMENT

Each meditation includes suggestions for further reading, listening, or action: Scriptures, prayers, music. Playlists for the songs may be found at www.elizabethturnage.com/ TheWaitingRoom.

FOR REFLECTION

At the end of each meditation, you will find a question for reflection and journaling.

APPENDIX

Here you will find additional helps to bring peace as you wait: further reading, exercises, playlists, and links to verses to color.

Your Only Comfort

For we don't live for ourselves or die for our-
selves. If we live, it's to honor the Lord. And if
we die, it's to honor the Lord. So whether we
live or die, we belong to the Lord.
ROMANS 14:7-8, NLT

AS I WAITED in a dimly-lit hospital hallway for our son to finish his first MRI—the one that followed the incidental discovery of a "something" on his brain, my mind turned to the first
question from the Heidelberg Catechism:

"What is your only comfort in life and in death?"[2]

I had pondered the answer just days before our son was
diagnosed with a brain tumor. A slew of family members had
suffered illness and loss: my mother, my father-in-law, and my
uncle had all suffered significant health issues. As I prayed that
the Lord would comfort my family members, I recalled the
Heidelberg's proclamation of hope, based on Romans 14:7-8:

"My only comfort in life and in death is that I am not my
own but belong to my faithful Savior Jesus Christ."[3]

How odd it seems at first that comfort comes from knowing
that we don't belong to ourselves. In the twenty-first century,
much emphasis is placed on our autonomy. We are taught to

value the idea of not being owned or directed by anyone.

And yet, as the apostle Paul explains in Romans 14:7, the assurance that we belong to the Lord eases our fears about life and death. Written into our very being is the basic need to belong. The good news of the gospel is that we *do belong* to a faithful and loving Savior who suffered so that we might have new life and eternal life. In Christ, whether we live or die, we honor the Lord. This reality brings us peace and comfort as we live in the uncertainty of the waiting room.

PRAYER

Lord, you are a loving and good Father who has claimed us as your own. Thank you for giving us your comfort as we wait—the knowledge that we and our precious ones belong to our faithful Savior Jesus Christ. Help us to be confident that whether we live or die, we do so for your glory. May that knowledge bring surpassing peace. In the name of your Son who died for us we pray, AMEN.

FURTHER ENCOURAGEMENT

- Read 1 Corinthians 6:19-20; Job 12:10; Acts 17:27-28.
- Read Heidelberg Catechism, Question One; please see Appendix.

FOR REFLECTION

What brings you comfort as you endure this wait?

You Are Forgiven

In him we have redemption through his blood,
the forgiveness of sins, in accordance with the
riches of God's grace…
EPHESIANS 1:7, NIV

ONE DAY, in the waiting room of my Dad's oncologist, I happened to sit next to an (annoying) angel. The very word *angel* in the Greek indicates a *messenger*, and this unlikely angel had a message from God for me and my dad.

My dad, who was now immobilized by tumors in his hips, was sitting in a wheelchair facing me. He chose this particular time and place to reveal a crucial piece of information he had previously withheld: his oral chemo pill was no longer defeating the cancer from the prostate, and he had stopped all treatment.

In that moment, I felt undone by rage at my powerlessness to help my dad, so I left my chair and walked to the edge of the crowded waiting room in an effort to calm myself. When I returned, I said quietly to my dad, "You did not tell me the truth when I asked. You told me you were 'tiptop.'"

He began to make excuses, to explain that he was only thinking of me and the burden I was carrying. I cut him off:

"You should have told me."

At this point the angel entered the story. A sturdy, middle-aged woman, she sat stuffed in the pleather chair connected to mine. Suddenly I felt a pat on my shoulder and heard her speak in a rough, country voice, "It'll be okay."

She continued, "Just so long as you know where you're going, it's all okay."

I nodded and looked pointedly at my dad, who frequently fought me on this point. I still wasn't sure if he was a Christian.

She repeated her message, "Just so long as you know you're saved. Jesus makes it all okay."

My dad turned back to me and repeated his apology. "I'm sorry." No excuses this time.

I still couldn't look him in the eye. I said, "It's okay. You're forgiven. I just wish you had told me."

The angel in the waiting room was right, even if I wasn't eager at first to hear her message. That day, both my dad and I needed the comforting knowledge of Ephesians 1:7, the knowledge that Jesus shed actual blood so that we might be forgiven.

I needed forgiveness for my unkindness to my dad. Dad needed a Savior to take the burden of guilt he had carried over a lifetime of unconfessed sin. As the angel had assured us, it would all be "okay" if we believed Jesus' ultimate sacrifice for us.

PRAYER

Precious Lord Jesus, thank you for shedding your
blood for us, for bearing God's wrath on my behalf.
Thank you for lifting the burden of our guilt from us.

Help us to live and love in the freedom of your forgiveness, AMEN.

FURTHER ENCOURAGEMENT

- Read 1 Peter 1:18; 1 John 1:7; 2:2.

- Listen to "Forgiveness" by Matthew West at https://
  youtu.be/oIbCpy0CQEo

FOR REFLECTION

In what ways do you and/or your loved one need to know
forgiveness in this season?

NOTES

Becoming Mature and Complete

Consider it pure joy, my brothers and
sisters, whenever you face trials of many kinds,
because you know that the testing of your faith
produces perseverance. Let perseverance finish
its work so that you may be mature and
complete, not lacking anything.
JAMES 1:2-4, NIV

ON THE FIRST day of August, I had jotted a note in my prayer journal under our son's name: "humility and gratitude." It's not that he isn't generally a humble and grateful twenty-two-year-old—but really, what twenty-two-year-old couldn't stand to grow in this area? (Or what fifty-two-year-old couldn't grow a little more, for that matter?)

This practice was nothing new; it's what I do. I anticipate or observe character issues in my children, and I begin asking God to work on it. But when our son was diagnosed with a brain tumor two days later, I wanted to take my prayer back. I prayed something like this:

> In the first place, God, I didn't want him to have
> to **suffer** to gain this humility and gratitude. In the

second place, God, **I** didn't want to have to suffer in order for my son to grow more mature. In the third place, I didn't really **mean** that prayer.

But God firmly showed me that there were no "take-backs" on this prayer; furthermore, perhaps there were some areas of *my* character that could benefit from such a trial. God wasn't content to let me remain unchanged. Instead, he was committed to my sanctification.

Sanctification is a big theological word that refers to the process by which God makes his children more like their Savior Jesus: more holy, more mature, more complete. Of the many lessons Scripture teaches about sanctification, two lessons in particular apply here:

1. God saves us with the purpose of making us more like his Son.

2. Whether we like it or not, God often uses suffering to help us grow and mature.

I am a feeble and sinful parent, but I still scribbled a prayer in my journal because I wanted our son to be mature and complete, lacking nothing. God did not scribble when he engraved my name into his hand. He nailed his Son to the cross and wrote my name with Jesus' blood. Such are the lengths to which our faithful Father has gone to make us, his precious children, mature and complete, lacking nothing.

PRAYER

Heavenly and faithful Father, we praise you for being the best Father. Please use this season of affliction in our lives to grow proven character in us. May this proven character in turn help us to hope as we wait. And may this hope not be disappointed, but find its fulfillment as we become more like you, AMEN.

FURTHER ENCOURAGEMENT

Read Romans 5:3-5; 2 Thessalonians 1:3-12.

FOR REFLECTION

Have you ever prayed a prayer you wanted to "take back"? How did God answer that prayer?

NOTES

4

God Rules Everything

Are not two sparrows sold for a penny?
Yet not one of them will fall to the ground
apart from the will of your Father. And
even the very hairs of your head are all
numbered. So don't be afraid; you are
worth more than many sparrows.
MATTHEW 10:29-31, NIV

FOUR DAYS AFTER our son's first MRI, we sat in an exam room, waiting to meet the neurosurgeon who would perform his brain surgery. As the clock ticked away, my mind ticked with it. Suddenly, a horrible thought occurred to me—OH NO, HIS HAIR!

Some boys are fine with the just-got-out-of-bed look for their hair, but our youngest son has never been like that. His siblings may have teased him during his teen years about his hair products, but they had to admit that his hair always looked awesome. Picturing our precious twenty-two-year-old with a shaved head, I felt yet another gut-punch of loss.

I did what I always do when I feel sad and completely powerless: I began to pray.

In the next few days, some words from the first Heidelberg

Catechism question came back to me:

> He also preserves me in such a way
> that without the will of my heavenly Father
> not a hair can fall from my head;
> indeed, all things must work together
> for my salvation.[4]

These words refer to God's gracious sovereignty. Unfortunately, many detractors have made a mockery of the biblical concept of God's sovereignty. Some view God as a dark warlord ruling over his people with cruel force; others portray him as a crazy-faced puppeteer jerking his little minions around with wild glee.

As Jesus explained to his disciples, God's sovereignty is reason to rejoice and praise: the Lord watches over us as a kind Father who cares compassionately for his children (Matthew 10). The Lord preserves and protects those in his care, and his will is for our good and for his glory.

It brought me great comfort to know that "not a hair would fall" from my son's head without the Lord willing it. In the sometimes-painful or humiliating experience of the waiting room, the Lord is changing us into people who more fully resemble him in love and compassion. Take comfort, friend, in the assurance that God rules everything.

PRAYER

Father God, we thank you for faithfully preserving us and so carefully watching over us. Please comfort us as we wait in the hope that this hard story is written by your loving hand. Help us to see you reigning as King over our lives; draw us to serve you more faithfully. In Jesus' ruling name, we pray, AMEN.

FURTHER ENCOURAGEMENT

- Read Psalm 11:4; Psalm 93:5; Psalm 97; Psalm 99.
- Listen to "O Worship the King" by Chris Tomlin at https://youtu.be/We9aR22C9BI.

FOR REFLECTION

How can you see God authoring this hard story for his glory and your good?

NOTES

5

Don't Panic—He's Got You

*Don't panic. I'm with you. There's no
need to fear for I'm your God. I'll give
you strength. I'll help you. I'll hold you
steady, keep a firm grip on you.*
ISAIAH 41:10, MSG

ON AN ORDINARY day in August, our son went for a routine sinus Cat-scan; that same day we learned that my father-in-law would need open heart surgery. My husband flew off to be with his parents. Shortly after 2 p.m., my mother-in-law texted to say my father-in-law's surgery had gone well.

A few minutes later, I was in my car when my husband called. I assumed he was just checking in, but his voice quaked as he asked me, "Are you at home?" When I told him I was almost home, his voice broke as he instructed, "Call me when you get there."

Immediately, panic rose, and I cried out in an unfamiliar, squeaky voice, "What's wrong? Your Dad?!— but—your mom just texted me that he's okay." My husband, a generally imperturbable man, was clearly crying as he repeated his request, "Just call me when you get home." Now I wailed. "Noooooo… What's WRONG??? IS IT ONE OF THE KIDS? I've pulled over. You can't do this to me. You have to tell me NOW!!!" Our son's Cat-scan didn't even enter my mind.

His voice broke, sobs escaping, as he told me. "The ENT called. They found something on [our son]'s CT. He has a— **mass.**" That heavy blob of a word that just sits on your chest with the weight of all its awful possibility.

Panic assaulted me. I felt my face go numb, while my body zinged with adrenaline. My heart felt like it was sizzling on a hot griddle; my stomach wound itself into a tangle of knots.

Denial quickly tried to push panic aside: *That can't be. I just saw him, and he's fine.*

My husband gently instructed me to go home and take our son to the hospital for an MRI.

And that's when it arrived. A quiet, almost eerie peace.

During a health crisis, it's normal to experience panic. The good news of the Bible is that God is neither shocked nor surprised by our wild-eyed fear. One of the most oft-written commands from the Lord to his people is, "Do not be afraid." These words acknowledge that we *will* feel fear—terror, panic, horror, dread—in this fallen world.

As we wait, what we desperately need is to be held. The Bible insists almost to the point of redundancy that our God is a stable God: he does not quake, shake, or tremble. Our firmly-fixed Lord, the very One who created the cosmos, has an unflinching grip on us.

PRAYER

Strong-gripped Father, we thank you that when we tremble in fear of earthly terrors, you hold us tight. Please, we pray, replace panic with peace in our

quivering hearts. We worship you as our unshakeable
King. May we be rooted in this truth in our hearts,
AMEN.

FURTHER ENCOURAGEMENT

- Read Psalm 55:1-8; 16-20; Philippians 4:5-7; Hebrews
  4:28-29.

- Listen to "Refuge" by Susan Calderazzo at https://vimeo.
  com/232853172.

FOR REFLECTION

What symptoms of panic have you experienced during this
time of crisis? Write them down and ask God to heal you and
help you when panic arises.

NOTES

6

How to Pray

Is anyone among you in trouble?
Let them pray. Is anyone happy?
Let them sing songs of praise.
JAMES 5:13, NIV

FOR MANY, the gut response when facing a stint in the waiting room is prayer. But how do we find words and concentration to pray in such times? I am easily distractible, so I write the essence of my prayers in a journal using an acronym I learned in high school: ACTS.

ACTS STANDS FOR:

> **A**doration: praising God for who he is and what he has done.
> **C**onfession: telling God the truth about your sins.
> **T**hanksgiving: thanking God for his salvation, for how he has already worked redemption.
> **S**upplication: asking God for help for yourself or others.

I gather words from a Psalm, going through one per day to give voice to my adoration of God. Early on the morning of August 4, I pulled out my prayer journal. It was the day after our son had the CT-Scan and the MRI that revealed a lesion on his brain; it was the day we were going to an appointment with the local neurosurgeon. I read from Psalm 42, then wrote this prayer, capitalizing certain words for emphasis:

> **A:** We pant for YOU, oh GOD. YOU are LIVING. YOU quench thirst—our SAVIOR and our GOD. We put our HOPE in YOU, GOD—we will yet PRAISE YOU!
>
> **C:** I am TEMPTED to ask WHY—to be AFRAID.
>
> **T:** I feel my heart so GUARDED—I feel PEACE that surpasses all UNDERSTANDING [from Phil. 4:6-8]—I have HOPE…"Though he slay me, yet will I trust in HIM." [from Job 13:15].
>
> **S:** LORD, PLEASE, PLEASE—Save our son—Heal this 'lesion,' shrink it, disappear it!

In this world, many well-meaning people will tell you they are "sending positive thoughts your way." I believe these positive thoughts are God's common grace to those who have not yet discovered the power, joy, and simplicity of prayer.

Prayer does not have to be eloquent, and we don't even have to come up with the words to pray. It so happened that the day I wrote this prayer, my "Psalm calendar" led me to Psalm 42, which includes these words:

> Why are you cast down, O my soul,
> and why are you in turmoil within me?
> Hope in God, for I shall again praise him,
> My salvation and my God (Psalm 42:5, ESV).

As you can see, in parts of my prayer, I quoted from some other verses in Scripture, which the Holy Spirit brought to my mind. It may be hard to find the words to pray as you wait, but using this simple guideline along with Psalms and other Scriptures may help.

PRAYER

Lord, we want to pray, but sometimes as we wait, we confess we don't feel like praying. Lead us to your Word which will guide us in adoring you, confessing our sins to you, thanking you, and asking you for what we need. Lead us to hope in you yet again even when our souls are in turmoil. In the name of your praying Son, our Savior, we ask, AMEN.

FURTHER ENCOURAGEMENT

- Read Psalm 42; Ephesians 6:18; Jeremiah 29:12.
- Listen to "My Help, My God" by Sandra McCracken at https://sandramccracken.bandcamp.com/track/my-help-my-god-psalm-42.

FOR REFLECTION

Try writing out a prayer using the ACTS acronym.

NOTES

7

Knowledge That Will Change Your World

Thus says the Lord, your Redeemer,
who formed you from the womb:
'I am the Lord, who made all things,
who alone stretched out the heavens,
who spread out the earth by myself....'
ISAIAH 44:24, ESV

"Knowledge that will change your world..."
IT IS A BRILLIANT tagline for a hospital. I first noticed it on a sticker in the parking deck of the medical center. It plays right into our deepest fears and fiercest desires in the season of a health crisis. I do not fault the hospital for using it. Instead, I thank them for the hope it offered us.

After all, many of the world's experts were gathered at this medical center, and they knew (almost) everything there was to know about brain tumors. Our neurosurgeon operated exclusively on brain tumors. He had performed thousands of awake craniotomies. Surely these people had the knowledge that would change our son's world.

And yet...I recognize my own idolatry in that way of thinking. Idols are things we trust in more than God to deliver us. Long ago, I heard a speaker suggest we uncover our idols by asking, "Where do you find your security, significance, and sense of safety?" As we played the waiting game, I would have had to confess, "I am seeking my sense of security and safety in these world-expert doctors."

The Bible warns us about putting our trust in idols, in earthly things that do not really have the power to save us. Isaiah 44 describes foolish people who take a piece of wood, use half of it to make a fire and the other half to carve an idol. They fall down before the idol and worship it, saying, "Rescue me… you are my god" (Isaiah 44:17, NLT). But the idol neither blinks nor moves, for it is merely a piece of wood. Isaiah observes, "The poor, deluded fool feeds on ashes. He trusts something that can't help him at all" (Isaiah 44:20, NLT).

Please don't misunderstand me—I do believe doctors and medical experts have much knowledge and skill to offer us. Still, the gospel invites us to trust fully in the one, true GOD who can and **will** deliver us, the God who made all things and knows all things. God, who has the knowledge that will truly change our world, invites us to come to him and rest in him.

PRAYER

All-knowing, ever-loving Father, you are our Creator and Redeemer. You know us fully, and one day we will fully know you and fully trust you. Thank you for the knowledge you have given to medical personnel and their faithfulness in acquiring it. Help us to trust in your knowledge more than theirs. In the name of your redeeming Son, our Savior, AMEN.

- Read Isaiah 43:9-20; Proverbs 3:5-6.

- Listen to "He Is God" by Susan Calderazzo at https://www.reverbnation.com/susancalderazzo/songs.

FOR REFLECTION

In what things are you looking for a sense of security, safety and significance during this season?

8

God Knows You

For now we see in a mirror dimly, but then
face to face. Now I know in part; then I shall
know fully, even as I have been fully known.
1 CORINTHIANS 13:12, ESV

THE STRESS, uncertainty, and waiting that you experience during a health crisis may make you feel as if you no longer know yourself. One minute you may be surprised at your kindness to a stranger, the next you may be shocked at your meanness to a loved one. You may find yourself amazed one moment at God-given patience, then struggling an hour later not to scream at a nurse who hasn't brought the painkiller yet. Take heart—such wild swings in emotions are fairly common during a health crisis.

While the theologian and pastor Dietrich Bonhoeffer was imprisoned by the Nazis during World War II, he wrote about this sense of not knowing himself in his poem, "Who Am I?" In the first several stanzas, he reports how others describe him: calm, cheerful, friendly, clear. Then he asserts with brutal honesty how he often sees himself:

Or am I only what I myself know of myself?

Restless and longing and sick, like a bird in a cage,
struggling for breath, as though hands were
compressing my throat,
yearning for colors, for flowers, for the voices of birds,
thirsting for words of kindness, for neighborliness,
tossing in expectation of great events,
powerlessly trembling for friends at an infinite distance,
weary and empty at praying, at thinking, at making,
faint, and ready to say farewell to it all?

His conclusion points us to the basis of our hope:

"Who I really am, you know me, I am yours, O God!"[5]

Bonhoeffer's hope was not rooted in his knowledge of himself. His circumstances had broken that sense of self. But he had hope because he was known fully by God. And that God who knew him when he did not know himself owned him fully and loved him in the midst of his sorrow.

God's knowledge of us offers unspeakable comfort. Isaiah assures us that God knows us by name; this intimate knowledge leads him to protect us when we pass through roaring waters or walk through the fire (Isaiah 43:1-3). Hosea writes that because God knows us, he remains near to us as we wander in the wilderness. (Hosea 13:4-5). The gospel gives us hope that though we may lose ourselves as we wait, God never loses us.

PRAYER

Lord, I confess that I feel crazy, not-myself, in this waiting season. Thank you, praise you, for knowing me fully—my sins, my weaknesses, my mood swings—and loving me faithfully. You say you are like a mother hen longing to wrap your chicks under your strong, sheltering wings. Let me take refuge there. In the knowledge of our Savior Jesus Christ I pray, AMEN.

FURTHER ENCOURAGEMENT

- Read Psalm 103:13-14; Isaiah 43:1-2; Nahum 1:7-8; Luke 13:34.

- Listen to "Be Still My Soul/I Will Rest" by Kari Jobe at https://www.youtube.com/watch?v=Tw2ep0t4zG8

FOR REFLECTION

How have you felt "not yourself" during this season? Hear God speaking his love over you just as you are in your grief.

9

Live by Every Word

*Yes, he humbled you by letting you go hungry
and then feeding you with manna, a food
previously unknown to you and your ancestors.
He did it to teach you that people do not live
by bread alone; rather we live by every word
that comes from the mouth of the Lord.*
DEUTERONOMY 8:3, NLT

ANYONE WHO HAS spent much time in the waiting room knows the humbling that comes during a health crisis. Stripped of the familiarities on which we often depend for comfort, we learn that we do not, in fact, live by bread alone.

The profound hope of Deuteronomy 8:3 is that God did not merely humble his people, but he also fed them. He fed them physically with something called *manna*, a word that in the original Hebrew literally means, "What's this?" It was a food unlike anything the Israelites had ever heard of, seen, or tasted. It fell from the sky, and it looked something like Frosted Flakes but was a lot more nutritious!

God fed his people physically with this strange food, and he fed them spiritually with his Word. As we do our time in the wilderness of waiting, we are humbled, and our hunger and thirst for good news intensifies. More precisely, more powerfully than any IV fluid, God's Word drips into our hearts and minds to slake our thirst, to energize us with the faith, hope, and love we desperately need.

- Our faith grows strong muscles as we drink in the stories of miraculous deeds God has already done, such as

  - o plastering the land of unbelieving Egypt with frogs (Exodus 8:2).
  - o knocking down a city wall with trumpet blasts (Joshua 6:1-6, 20).

- Our hope is fattened up as we eagerly digest words like, "This is a spiritual refining process, with glory just around the corner" (1 Peter 4:13, MSG).

- Our love is energized to flow outward as we taste the goodness of the Lord's delight over us and the comfort of his nearness to us:

"The LORD your God is in your midst,
    a mighty one who will save;
he will rejoice over you with gladness;
    he will quiet you by his love;
he will exult over you with loud singing"
    (Zephaniah 3:17, ESV).

Throughout our journey in the waiting room, I was often asked about my apparent calm. I could only explain it by pointing to three essentials: prayer, The Word, and community.

Dear friends, take up and read this marvelous Word; you

will find there the sustenance you intensely crave.

PRAYER

Lord, we thank you for feeding us what we most desperately need—your Word. Not only did you provide the Scriptures, but you made the Word flesh, and you sent Jesus to dwell among us. Help us by your Spirit to meet Jesus in your Living Word day by day, moment by moment, AMEN.

FURTHER ENCOURAGEMENT

- Read Deuteronomy 30:11-14; Romans 10:8-10.
- Listen to "The Word Is So Near" by Michael Card at https://youtu.be/biXrKOaIJq4

FOR REFLECTION

What verses have encouraged your faith, hope, and love during this season? Write them out in a journal, on a card, or on a note app on your phone.

NOTES

10

Your Troubled Heart

Let not your hearts be troubled;
believe in God; believe also in me.
JOHN 14:1, ESV

IN PREPARATION FOR his first brain surgery, our son had to have a Functional-MRI. In this exam, the patient is asked to do certain activities while their brain function is measured. The F-MRI, as it is called, offers crucial mapping of the brain, showing what areas the tumor might affect; it guides the surgeon's surgical plan. Before taking our son back for the MRI, the tech told me the procedure would take around two hours.

It was God's kindness that got John 14:1 stuck in my head, here at the beginning of this strange and frightening journey. Jesus spoke these powerful and hopeful words to his disciples at the Last Supper, the night before his death. Peter had just uttered his famous declaration that he would *never* deny Jesus, and Jesus had asked him poignantly, "Will you lay down your life for me?" Jesus then gave Peter the startling prediction, "Truly, truly I tell you, the rooster will not crow till you have denied me three times" (John 13:37-38, ESV).

Jesus knew the suffering that he and his disciples would soon face. He also recognized that Peter and the other disciples could not fully comprehend the journey that lay before them. In John 14-17, Jesus prepared their hearts with many instructions and truths that they would only later understand.

As the waiting area clock ticked off two hours, I began to get fidgety. *When* would they bring our son back? I began to draw the words:

LET NOT YOUR HEARTS BE TROUBLED.

Two and a half hours. How much longer can he endure?

BELIEVE IN GOD.

Two hours and 45 minutes. Time dragged on; the waiting room emptied; a tech finally emerged at three hours to say they were almost done…

BELIEVE ALSO IN ME.

To *believe,* according to Merriam-Webster, is "to have a firm conviction about the goodness, efficacy, or ability of something."[6]

Did I have a firm conviction about God's "goodness, efficacy, or ability"? Yes. I believed that God redeems the very worst evil (Genesis 50:20).

Did I have a firm conviction about Christ's goodness? Yes. Though he was God, he suffered the very worst of humiliations: being beaten, mocked, betrayed, and hung on a cross, for *my* sins.

My heart was troubled as I thought of the misery our son was enduring. I hated it for him. And yet I believed in God; I also believed in Jesus. I knew we might have to wait to see it, but one day redemption would come.

PRAYER

Redeeming God, thank you for your Word which reminds us of how you faithfully loved Jesus and his disciples through their worst days. Sustaining God, thank you for drawing our troubled hearts to trust in your goodness on our worst days. In Jesus' suffering name we pray, AMEN.

FURTHER ENCOURAGEMENT

- Read John 13:36-John 14:7.
- Listen to "Sweet Comfort" by Sandra McCracken, at https://sandramccracken.bandcamp.com/album/psalms

FOR REFLECTION

Choose one of the verses listed above to draw or doodle. As you draw, meditate on the truth of these words.

NOTES

11

Sharing the Story

I will teach you hidden lessons from our past—
stories we have heard and known,
stories our ancestors handed down to us.
PSALM 78:2-3, NLT

"Transform this horrible story into a display of YOUR GLORY."

I PENNED THESE WORDS in my prayer journal on the morning we planned to tell our other three children and their spouses about our son's diagnosis. Along this journey, there were bad days, there were good days, and there were the worst days. This was one of the worst days.

I dreaded sharing the news. We knew that the moment our kids heard the words, "Your brother has been diagnosed with a brain tumor," they would feel the extraordinary pain of suffering with a loved one. My only hope was the prayer I had written, that the Lord would "transform this story into a display of his glory."

The Bible insists that even the worst stories must be remembered because as we recall and retell them, we will be led to follow and worship God. The Israelites told their good stories,

39

the stories of how God rescued them (Exodus 15:1-18), and their bad ones, of days in battle when they turned around and ran in fear from their enemy (Psalm 78:8-11). They believed that in all of these stories the Lord's faithfulness, the Lord's graciousness, and the Lord's holiness, shone through. They believed that in sharing these stories of God's goodness, their faith and hope in the Lord grew.

Dan Allender and Tremper Longman, in their excellent book on the Psalms, *Cry of the Soul*, describe hope as a "vision of redemption in the midst of decay."[7] In our family, we have a saying about terrible or terrifying stories that captures this hope: "This will make a really good story one day."

On that day, we did not know what that really good story would be, but because of Jesus, we had hope that it would come. Today I can tell you some good stories that came from this terrible story, stories of a family coming together to support one another, stories of the exquisite sacrifices our son's twenty-something siblings made on behalf of their brother. And yet, as someone who is still waiting for Jesus to come and restore all broken things, I believe God will bring even more glory from this story one day.

PRAYER

Story-writing God, author of every moment of our lives, we praise you for your faithfulness. We ask that you give us eyes to see "a vision of redemption" in the midst of our worst-day stories. Please continue to transform horrible stories into a display of your glory. In Jesus' healing and hopeful name we pray, AMEN.

- Read Psalm 78; Psalm 145.

- Listen to "Add to the Beauty" by Sara Groves at https://youtu.be/9htYsEbIADU

FOR REFLECTION

Tell or write a story of a time that God transformed a "worst-day story" into something beautiful.

12

Prayer Requests:
Inviting Community to Pray

I urge you, first of all, to pray for all people.
Ask God to help them; intercede on their
behalf, and give thanks for them.
1 TIMOTHY 2:1, NLT

PRAYING FOR ONE ANOTHER is one way we can bear one another's burdens; it also powerfully reveals the interdependence of the body of Christ. Before our son was diagnosed with a brain tumor, I confess sometimes I hesitated to mention prayer requests through more public vehicles like church prayer chains. In our season in the waiting room, though, I discovered that there are many good reasons to invite community to pray.

1. **The Bible tells us that both Jesus (Romans 8:34; Hebrews 7:25) and the Holy Spirit (Romans 8:26) are interceding for us.** If two of the three persons of the Holy Trinity are praying for us, then Christian community should do likewise.

2. **It allows others to be a part of the answer to your**

prayer. For example, I asked our church to pray for community for our son while he was back home during this year of surgeries. He had been away at college for four years, so he had few close friends remaining in our town. The church responded by praying *and* offering fellowship. One man took him to lunch on several occasions, a group of grad students invited him to join a book club, and others encouraged him to join the college and career Bible study.

3. **It relieves us of our emotional burden and our isolation.** Eugene Peterson writes that praying in community is essential. Doing so, he says, "defends us against the commonest diseases of prayer: the tyranny of our emotions, the isolationism of our pride."[8] Praying alone, especially during times of crisis, can lead to emotional exhaustion; limited vision can cause us to lose hope. A praying community helps us see beyond our individual story to what God is doing in his kingdom.

4. **Other people's prayers envelop us as a comforting quilt of hope and help.** Hear the words sent to me by a dear friend who has a gift for writing prayers:

"Please protect [Elizabeth's son] and family from the evil one and discouragement of any kind. Please lift them all up on Your wings to 'soar as eagles' (Is. 40:31), for they hope in You. Please be glorified in all aspects of this treatment and continue to bless them with unity and precious relationships together. Through Your Spirit, please fill them to overflowing with Your love, and enable them to be a glorious witness of Your supernatural grace to all who interact with them, for Your glory. Bless them, dear Abba, for they put their trust in You alone."[9]

Dear friend, do not go it alone in this hard season. Invite others to pray for you; you will bless others even as they bless you.

PRAYER

Lord, please humble us. Help us to cry "help," to invite others to bear our burdens. Thank you for your church, the body of believers, who join us in our suffering through prayer. In Jesus' praying name we pray, AMEN.

FURTHER ENCOURAGEMENT

- Read 1 Thessalonians 5:14; James 5:13-16.

- Listen to "Come People of the Risen King" by Keith and Kristyn Getty and Stuart Townend at https://store.getty-music.com/us/song/come-people-of-the-risen-king/

FOR REFLECTION

In what ways have you been strengthened by others' prayers during this season?

13

Looking for a Better Place

But they were looking for a better place,
a heavenly homeland. That is why God
is not ashamed to be called their God,
for he has prepared a city for them.
HEBREWS 11:16, NLT

WHEN OUR SON was diagnosed with a brain tumor, he, and we, wrestled with the agonizing possibility that he might lose his hope and dream of getting his master's degree in vocal performance, of singing sacred music in ways that would transport listeners to another world. While there is nothing wrong with having hopes and dreams in this life, we as Christians must always stake our deepest longings in the world to come, the "better place," the "heavenly homeland."

Hebrews 11, sometimes called the "Hall of Faith," begins by defining faith as "the assurance of things hoped for, the conviction of things not seen" (Hebrews 11:1, ESV). It continues with stories of people living this faith; among the ones mentioned are Noah, David, Rahab, Sarah, and of course Abraham. Of those who walked by faith, trusting in God's promises, some enjoyed the fulfillment of God's promises in this life: some "overthrew kingdoms;" others "shut the mouths of lions" (Hebrews 11:32, NLT). Abraham and Sarah, despite several significant stumbles along the way, received the promised child, whom they named Isaac ("laughter"), to emphasize the joy of their faith fulfilled.

And yet, the author of Hebrews reminds us that not all of the faithful see all of God's promises fulfilled in their lifetime. Abraham and Sarah lived in tents outside of the Promised Land (Hebrews 11:9); Moses was not allowed to enter the Promised Land (Numbers 20:12). Many of those named in the Hebrews Hall of Faith suffered violent deaths and torture; others were imprisoned, "oppressed and mistreated" (Hebrews 11:35b-38, NLT). One thing is clear; all who walk by faith will endure suffering along the way.

From these faith journeys, we learn at least two things that can encourage us as we wait:

1. We must keep our eyes fixed on the "better place," the "heavenly homeland" which awaits us. When we draw our identity and sense of life from things in this world, focusing on the highs and lows of our present circumstances, we will find ourselves tossed about. But when our eyes are fixed on the hope of our identity in Christ, and the ultimate reward that he has secured for us, we will walk toward home with sure and steady steps.

2. The suffering we endure keeps us looking and longing for the better place. As Nancy Guthrie writes, "There is something better, somewhere better, Someone better... than any thing, any place, any person who has captured our devotion in the here and now. It is real. And it is forever."[10]

As you wait, dear friends, run by faith alongside the great cloud of witnesses which has gone before you, fixing your eyes on Jesus, the author and perfecter of your faith (Hebrews 12:1-2). You will soon see him, and he will welcome you home.

PRAYER

God, forgive us when we fix our eyes only on the things of this earth. Help us, as we wait, to remember that we are strangers here, but we will one day be at home with you. In Jesus' faithful name we place our hope and find our peace, AMEN.

FURTHER ENCOURAGEMENT

- Read Hebrews 11:1-12:2.

- Listen to "I Can Only Imagine" by Mercy Me at https://youtu.be/Rlu-a1lgeTo.

FOR REFLECTION

Do you have earthly hopes in which you invest a lot of time and energy? Spend some time "looking for that better place" in prayer. What sweet joys will you experience there?

NOTES

14

Our Ultimate Question

For the thing that I fear comes upon me,
and what I dread befalls me.
JOB 3:25, ESV

I WAS IMMERSED in a sweet season of shalom when my daily Bible reading landed me in the book of Job. Our eldest daughter was planning her wedding to her beloved; our youngest son was giving final piano and voice recitals before graduating from college. Other children were in transition, preparing to go to graduate school, taking on exciting new roles in their careers. I myself was in the eager planning stages of retreats I would teach in coming months, and my husband, an orthopedic surgeon, was happily repairing torn up shoulders and knees.

This is why, as I read Job, I could not help but ask what felt like the book's ultimate question: "Lord, what if we experienced the kind of extreme loss, the inexplicable suffering that Job did? Would we still praise you? Would we still trust you?"

The Book of Job centers around this question: how should a believer respond to God in the midst of suffering? At the beginning of the account, God is the one who points Job out to Satan as an upright man; Satan counters that if Job lost everything, he would curse God and die. God gives Satan permission to inflict trials on Job, and by the end of Chapter 1, Job has lost all his children and all his property.

If that weren't bad enough, Job's wife and friends quickly turn on him. His wife, in her misery, urges Job to "curse God and die" (Job 2:9, ESV). His friends advise Job to confess the hidden sin that they are convinced has caused the suffering. Job refuses the counsel of both his wife and his friends, insisting on being honest with himself and with God.

Through most of the rest of the book, Job rants, Job raves, but he does not curse God. He curses the day he was born, but he does not curse God. He proclaims his innocence; he proclaims God's might, but he does not curse God. What Job wants most is to meet with God directly (Job 13:3). And indeed, as Eugene Peterson observes, "...perhaps that is what all of us who are suffering want—not a definitive explanation but a divine encounter."[11]

The beauty of Job's lament is its honesty and its result: he never fully loses hope in the goodness of God.

May we wrestle as Job did, and may we come to proclaim our answer with Job,

"Though he slay me, yet will I hope in him...." (Job 13:15, NIV).

PRAYER

Lord, help us we pray, in this season of extraordinary loss, to seek your face, to believe in your goodness. Meet us in this place, we beg, face to face. We do not ask for an explanation, but for a profound encounter of your presence. In Jesus' suffering name, we pray, AMEN.

- Read Job 1-2.

- Listen to "Though You Slay Me" by Shane and Shane at https://www.youtube.com/watch?v=qyUPz6_TciY.

FOR REFLECTION

What questions do you have about your suffering?

NOTES

15

God's Answer

*I know that my Redeemer lives, and that in
the end, he will stand on the earth.*
JOB 19:25, NIV

FINALLY, JOB GETS his wish (see "Our Ultimate Question")—
the Lord "answers" him out of the whirlwind (Job 38:1).
Picture the scene: here is Job, sore-ridden body, friend-beaten
emotions, sitting in the dust, still struggling to understand his
misery. Suddenly, a storm comes up, and out of something like
a tornado, "The Lord" begins to speak. (God's personal name,
Yahweh, translated *The Lord*, is used to emphasize his personal
presence.)

The Lord's answer for Job in the next four chapters includes
some seventy questions, beginning with this flattening stroke:

"Who is this that darkens counsel by words without knowledge? Dress for action like a man; I will question you, and you
will make it known to me" (Job 38:2-3, ESV).

And so it begins, as the Lord unfurls his majesty like a scroll
before Job. He trots out the stars he has chained together and
the calves whose births he has counted, the beasts he has sub-
dued, and the sea which he himself has boiled. When the Lord
pauses for Job's response, Job can only stammer, "Behold, I am

of small account; what shall I answer you? I lay my hand over my mouth" (Job 40:3-4, ESV).

The Lord's deluge of questions may seem heavy at first, but a second glance reveals a flood of love. The Lord's purpose is to floor Job, to lower him to an attitude of awe and humility. From that position, Job can fully recognize and receive the God-who-is-with-him in the storm. The Lord appeared before Job, not to defend himself or to explain Job's suffering, as Job had wished, but to give Job the supreme gift that we all most desperately crave even if we don't realize it: the gift of *himself.*

Indeed, in the end, Job discovers he was right all along: his Redeemer *does* live. After the Lord finishes his "answer," Job confesses, "I had heard of you by the hearing of the ear, but now my eye sees you" (Job 42:5, ESV). Although Job did not know Jesus as we do, in a very real way, he saw the shadow of Jesus' sufferings and the joy Jesus would bring.

In the Book of Job, God answers our deepest questions about inexplicable suffering. What we need, God says, is *not* an explanation, but presence, his presence. Job *believed* by faith that his Redeemer lived; we *know* that our Redeemer Jesus has lived, died, and been raised from the dead. We also know that one day he will return to restore us to the full presence of the Lord who waits to defeat all wickedness and end all suffering.

PRAYER

Lord, thank you for knowing what we most desperately need in this season of suffering—your presence. Thank you that you have come near to us in Jesus and that you have given us the Spirit as our Comforter until Jesus comes again. In Jesus' very present name we pray, AMEN.

- Read Job 38-42.

- Listen to "The Job Suite" by Michael Card at https://youtu.be/OuqOx3B4WY0.

FOR REFLECTION

What explanations have you longed for during this journey? In what ways have you experienced God's presence?

NOTES

16

Comfort as You Have Been Comforted

*Blessed be the God and Father of our Lord
Jesus Christ, the Father of mercies and God of
all comfort, who comforts us in all our afflictions, so that we may be able to comfort those
who are in any affliction, with the comfort
with which we ourselves are comforted by God.*
2 CORINTHIANS 1:3-4, ESV

MOST OF THE patients in Neuro-ICU have had strokes, trau-
matic brain injuries, or brain surgery; many are in critical condition. The Neuro-ICU waiting area teems with families and
friends of patients waiting for news or a brief window to see
their loved ones, possibly for the last time. Many camp out in
the area, not having the money for a hotel room, or not want-
ing to leave in case the patient's condition changes.

Because the small waiting area bathroom of the Neuro-ICU
serves many women and children, some of whom are using
sinks for sponge-baths and tooth-brushing, the housecleaning
staff can't always keep up with the cleaning needs. For this
reason, it can be a generally messy and depressing place.

On one of our happy days, a day when our son was doing
well enough to be released from the Neuro-ICU to the regular

Neuro floor, I made a visit to this unrestful restroom. As soon as I pushed open the door, I heard a loud wailing coming from the disabled-accessible stall. Glancing that way, I could see that a woman was crumpled on the floor.

I felt her ache keenly and wanted to comfort her. Should I go to her? Should I offer to pray for her? I decided to go to the bathroom and then decide. I sat in the stall praying for her, asking God to give me the courage to reach out. I wanted to say, "I've been there. At times, I've been so discouraged along this journey, so demoralized by the process that I wanted to curl up and cry on a bathroom floor. The only thing that kept me upright was a Holy Spirit spurt of hope that came at just the right time."

I never got up the nerve. I left the bathroom without saying a word. I had been comforted by the God of all comfort through the vast community of faith, and I did not share that comfort with a broken-hearted sister. I have always felt sad about that.

And yet—even as I consider my failure to offer comfort to my fellow traveler in the neuro-ICU bathroom, I recall the One who never fails to show compassion to the broken-hearted—our Lord Jesus. Once, a woman who had been bleeding for years touched him in the midst of a bustling crowd. Jesus noticed. He stopped and asked who had touched him. He wanted to see the face of the woman who was not only comforted but healed by his power. When she came forward, he spoke tender and strong words to her, "Daughter, your faith has made you well; go in peace" (Luke 8:42-48).

In this season, may we know Jesus' comfort spoken into our deepest agony as well as our darkest failures. In him, we shall find comforting peace.

PRAYER

Dear Lord, help us to see others' pain and to share the comfort we have known from you. Thank you for sending Jesus, who never fails to offer comfort to the hurting. Amen.

FURTHER ENCOURAGEMENT

Read 2 Corinthians 1:3-7; Romans 15:1-3.

FOR REFLECTION

Look around you today for someone who might need comfort. Say a prayer, say hello, offer a smile, or hold the elevator for them. Look for a glimpse of God's glory in the exchange.

17

I Know Whom I Have Believed

…for I know whom I have believed…
2 TIMOTHY 1:12, ESV

DURING OUR SON'S second brain surgery, the words, "I know whom I have believed" kept coming to mind. When I quoted this fragment of 2 Timothy in an email update to faithful prayer warriors, one gracious friend emailed back with the last part of the verse: "and I am convinced that he is able to guard until that Day what has been entrusted to me" (2 Tim. 1:12, ESV).

Our friend knew that we needed to hear the last part of this verse that Paul wrote from a prison cell. He begins by saying, "I know whom I have believed," expressing his firm faith in the God who has rescued in the past. In the second part, he expresses his confidence in the God who is trustworthy in the present and brings hope for the future. As we waited for news about our son, we needed to focus on the God who redeems past, present, and future.

Although Paul is talking about how God will guard the gospel entrusted to us, this passage also assures us that God is able to guard other precious things that he has entrusted to us.

Many years ago, in a fit of frustration with our pediatrician,

I declared my complete dependence on God to guard the children he had entrusted to me and my husband:

> Our pediatrician used to conclude **every** visit with a stern lecture: "Watch them. They will climb it, eat it, or stick it in their noses…." He would continue with his list of scenarios until he drove home his two major points: first, my children would find a way to endanger their lives, and second, **I** was responsible for preventing their self-destruction.
>
> One day, as a weary mom of four children aged six-months to six-years, I had lost all tact, so I responded bluntly to his lecture, "I will watch them, Dr. ---. But I am thankful that God is watching over them too, because if it were all up to me, none of them would have survived past six months." I may have said it with a hint of defensiveness, but the truth was sure: God had entrusted these children to me, but it was he who was guarding them and guiding them each day.

Whether we are watching our child get on the bus for the first time, bringing soup to our spouse when he or she is sick with the flu, or waiting for MRI results for our loved one, we can and must entrust them to God. He is the Creator, Redeemer and Sustainer.

In addition to reminding us of our present hope for our loved ones, 2 Timothy 1:12 also points us to the future hope we need to recall in the waiting room, the Day when Christ will return. Whatever happens, whether our son survives this health crisis or not, God is guarding him, and Jesus is coming back to take him—and us—home.

As the missionary Amy Carmichael wrote about the "peace-giving power" of 2 Timothy 1:12, "He is able. I know. I will trust."[12]

PRAYER

All-powerful, ever-faithful God, thank you for the confidence that you are able, and that we can trust in you in this frightening season. Help us to walk in faith, hope, and love until Jesus returns, AMEN.

FURTHER ENCOURAGEMENT

- Read 2 Timothy 1:8-14.

- Listen to "I Know Whom I Have Believed" by Antrite Mennonite Choir at https://www.youtube.com/watch?v=_bRV3J4n8cc.

FOR REFLECTION

Have you ever considered it **your** responsibility to safeguard the life of your loved one? Write a letter to God about entrusting him with the lives of those you love.

NOTES

18

Loss of Dignity

They divided my garments among them, and
for my clothing they cast lots.
JOHN 19:24, ESV

THROUGHOUT HIS LIFE, my dad sought to maintain a certain "decorum," as he would have called it. As an English professor, he not only chose his words precisely, he also dressed in a manner he thought fitting to his profession. To class, he wore a starched button down, Repp-striped-tie, blazer, and dress pants. Even in retirement, he had a classic daily uniform: heavy cotton polo shirt, khakis, and Bass lace-up tennis shoes.

It was shocking, then, as his health plummeted, to see him dressed in only a gray t-shirt and an adult diaper. As the pain increased from the tumors in his hips, the doctor had prescribed a fentanyl patch. Under the influence of the heavy narcotics, my father, a man who once enunciated every word clearly, began to slur his speech, fumbling to find the words to ask for a drink of water.

Humiliation often accompanies health crises. It is distressing to see our loved one stripped of dignity. Hospital gowns, bedside urinals, adult diapers, and shaved heads are just a few of the shameful losses patients may bear. As I cringed at my dad's suffering, an image came to mind: I pictured Jesus hanging on the cross with something resembling a bedsheet wrapped around his private parts and legs. Maybe you've seen a similar picture on a Good Friday church bulletin or on a stained-glass window.

When we experience the loss of dignity of a health crisis, we can take comfort in knowing that our Lord has suffered worse. Describing the humiliation of the crucifixion, Tony Reinke writes, "The clothes of Jesus were ripped off his body and divvied up. Hanging naked on a tree, Christ absorbed the unmitigated exposure to God's wrath—with no fig leaves, no animal skins, nothing to cover him. In his defenseless exposure to God's full wrath, he died for my sins and he turned the tables on Satan...."[13]

It is painful to watch our loved ones suffer; it is painful to consider the suffering Jesus bore for us. Still, Hebrews 12 encourages us to run the race with endurance, fixing our eyes on Jesus, who, "for the joy set before him endured the Cross, despising the shame." According to Hebrews 2:9-10, Christ was "crowned with glory and honor because of the suffering of death" (ESV). Take heart, dear friends: as your loved one suffers appalling indignities: Christ is preparing them—and you—for a life of eternal glory.

PRAYER

Precious Lord Jesus, as we gaze at you suffering on the Cross for our sins, we marvel at your love for us. When our loved ones suffer the indignities that come with declining health, help us to see the hope of glory. In your glorious name we pray, AMEN.

Read Hebrews 2:9-10; John 19:17-27.

FOR REFLECTION

Write a prayer naming all of the indignities you have witnessed or had to take part in during this season. Tell God the truth about how you feel. Ask him to reveal his glory in this suffering.

NOTES

19

Normal Grief

I am counted among those who go down to the pit; I am a man who has no strength....
PSALM 88: 4, ESV

MY DAD WAS actively dying, and our son had survived three surgeries and now was enduring a six-week course of IV antibiotics. I was done in. I pounded out my rage on the keys of my laptop, letter by letter, word by word, laying out my fury at the indignity of dying, my fury at my inability to prevent my loved ones' suffering. I shot the email to three dear friends who love me well; I knew I could trust them to hear my true heart and speak good counsel into my agony. They did, each in her own precious way.

The day after receiving my email rant, one of my dear friends called me. A gifted counselor, she gently asked, "You know all of the things you mentioned in your email—irrational anger, overindulging, exhaustion, irritability? You **do** know those are all characteristics of grief, right?" It was so sweet to hear her say that. Here I thought I was losing my mind, and she told me that given what we had been through, I was completely **normal**!

Psalm 88 does the same thing. You won't hear it quoted

often. It's pretty dark. But the Holy Spirit breathed it into God's Word for a reason. In a season of confusion and grief, as Dr. Carmen Imes, associate professor of Old Testament, writes, "we need the darker psalms—psalms that echo our own experiences of alienation and struggle; psalms willing to voice the questions we thought were off limits."[14]

Listen to some of the questions and accusations voiced by the Psalmist:

- "You have put me in the depths of the pit, in the regions dark and deep" (Psalm 88:6, ESV).

- "You have caused my companions to shun me; you have made me a horror to them." (Psalm 88:8, ESV).

- "Is your steadfast love declared in the grave, or your faithfulness in Abbadon?" (Psalm 88:11, ESV).

Heman, the author of Psalm 88, laments a friend's betrayal, not the losses of a health crisis; yet, his sense of being abandoned by God may feel familiar to those in the waiting room. Unlike many other Psalms of lament, Psalm 88 does not make a turn toward praising God at the end. Hear the last line:

"You have caused my beloved and my friend to shun me; My companions have become darkness" (Psalm 88:18, ESV).

Are faith and hope to be found in such a Psalm? Yes, indeed. Psalm 88 expresses strong faith, the faith to trust God with the dark emotions of grief and the questions that seem to have no answers. Psalm 88 also expresses powerful hope, the hope that God is listening, even if he has not yet answered. Dear friend, know that God awaits your cries of normal grief and stands ready to meet you in your confusion. One day soon, the wait will be over, and you will rest in his loving presence.

PRAYER

God of our salvation, we cry out to you in our grief, confusion and anger. Give rest, we plead, to our troubled souls. In Jesus' trustworthy name we ask, AMEN.

FURTHER ENCOURAGEMENT
Read Psalm 88 aloud.

FOR REFLECTION
What seemingly wild emotions of normal grief have you experienced? How does it make you feel to know these emotions are normal during such a time?

NOTES

(**20**)

Change of Plans

'For I know the plans I have for you,' says the
Lord. 'They are plans for good and not for
disaster, to give you a future and a hope.'
JEREMIAH 29:11, NLT

- I was planning to write a devotional or perhaps a book on how to keep a prayer journal.

- Our son was planning to move to Ithaca, NY to begin a master's program in vocal performance.

- My husband and I were planning to travel to New York City to celebrate our 35th anniversary.

BEFORE THE CT that changed everything, we had plans, and they weren't bad plans. But God had something different in mind. There is nothing like a health crisis to redirect our attention from our plans for life on this earth to God's plans for our eternal lives, starting…*now*. As eighty-eight-year-old J.I. Packer, renowned theologian, affirmed after learning that he had macular degeneration, "God knows what he's up to…. And I've had enough experiences of his goodness in all sorts of ways not to have any doubt about the present circumstances…. Some good, something for his glory, is going to come out of it."[15]

I'm afraid we too often quote Jeremiah 29:11 and its hopeful note of "plans for good, plans with a future and a hope" without considering the context in which it was written. The Israelites, God's people, have been exiled to Babylon from their home in Jerusalem after repeated disobedience and multiple warnings to repent. The Lord directs the Israelites to seek and pray for the welfare of Babylon, to build houses and marry and have children there, even as they wait for the Lord to return them to their home. The stint in Babylon was all part of God's greater plan to bless the Israelites and to bless the world.

Just as God planned redemption and restoration for the Israelites, he has worked his redemption plan for Christians. The plan is for our Christ-likeness to be magnified and for his gospel to be multiplied. If we trust in God's plan, we have hope when disaster apparently befalls us. We are to continue seeking his face, even in the exile of the waiting room. As we wait, we know that God is completing the good work that he has begun in us (Phil. 1:6), and that one day soon Christ will return and restore all broken things. Such are God's glorious plans for a future and a hope that we are looking forward to as we wait.

PRAYER

Lord, help us to understand that our plans too often focus on building "houses" here: careers, families, wealth. Your plans far exceed ours, as you are intent on building us into a temple, a people who glorify you in all that we are and all that we do. Thank you that you have a better plan for us, AMEN.

FURTHER ENCOURAGEMENT
Read Jeremiah 29:1-11; Philippians 1:6; and 1 John 3:2.

FOR REFLECTION
What plans of yours or a loved one have been disrupted by this season in the waiting room? Ask God to help you trust him to work his good plan in your life.

21

'Tis So Sweet to Trust in Jesus

So if you are suffering in a manner that pleases
God, keep on doing what is right, and trust
your lives to the God who created you,
for he will never fail you.
1 PETER 4:19, NLT

IN THE ELECTRIFIED atmosphere of the waiting room, music can soothe taut nerves as nothing else can. One hymn that spread peace through my fraught body as I waited was the simple and lovely piece, "'Tis So Sweet to Trust in Jesus."

Although I loved the hymn's lyrics, there was one line that always puzzled me:

> "Jesus, Jesus, how I trust him, how I've ***proved*** him o'er and o'er."

One thing I *knew* for sure—I had certainly *not* proved Jesus—*he* had in fact, proved himself *to me* "o'er and o'er." Finally, I looked up the word *prove* and discovered the archaic meaning: "to learn or find out by experience."[16] Now *that* made sense. Consider this sentence, not so pretty to sing, but easier to understand for contemporary minds:

"Jesus, Jesus, how I trust him, how I've **learned him, discovered by experience,** how trustworthy he is."

Louisa Stead, the author of the hymn, discovered through painful experience how very trustworthy Jesus was. On a lovely day at the beach in the late 1800's, she, her husband, and their four-year-old daughter were relaxing at the seashore. Suddenly they heard cries from the ocean—a young boy was floundering in the water. Louisa's husband attempted to save him, but both the boy and her husband ended up drowning. Louisa was left a widow with a young daughter and no financial resources.

One day, when she had nothing left to feed her daughter, she found a package on her front doorstep containing food and money. Out of her firsthand knowledge of Jesus' wondrous provision, Louisa Stead wrote the hymn, "'Tis So Sweet to Trust in Jesus."[17] Like Job, Louisa met with extreme loss and suffering. In her deepest pain, she came to know Jesus intimately.

In the waiting places, we have a similar opportunity to know Jesus as a precious lover and proven provider. This trustworthy Jesus beckons us to lean into his solid presence today. This trustworthy Jesus promises to be with us until the end, that day when he finally returns and we fully rest.

PRAYER

Jesus, precious Jesus, how you have proved yourself over and over. Even as I waver in my trust of you, you give me grace to trust you more. Thank you for being so very near in these trying days. In your trustworthy name we pray, AMEN.

- Read Ephesians 2:8; 1 Peter 4:12-19.

- Listen to "'Tis So Sweet to Trust in Jesus" by Casting Crowns at https://youtu.be/ZiEqKpN90W4.

FOR REFLECTION

How have you seen Jesus' wonderful provision in this hard season?

NOTES

22

When You Are Lonely

My God, My God,
why have you forsaken me?
MATTHEW 27:46.

DURING HIS BRAIN tumor/neuronal dysplasia odyssey, our son endured the worst of health procedures with incredible resolve and calm. But one of the earliest diagnostic nightmares, the Functional-MRI, left him looking like a de-stuffed dog toy after a sharp-toothed terrier got through with it.

After three and a half hours in that narrow tube, being asked to do things like raise his right hand or repeat a sentence like "the cow jumped over the moon," he limped out, collapsing into a chair near the elevator as soon as the tech left us. Lowering his head, he covered his face with his hands and sobbed. It was one of the rare times I saw him weep during this journey. Putting my hand on his shoulder, I asked if the procedure was painful. He shook his head and murmured, "Just so lonely."

Later, our son told us that his time in that MRI was the most isolating experience he had ever known. As he explained, "People will tell you how Jesus is always with you, but even Matt Chandler (the pastor of Village Church in Dallas) said that there were times that he did not feel Jesus' presence during his brain cancer journey."

Indeed, in this season of waiting there will be times when we feel utterly alone. In such moments, we can remember that Jesus really does know how we feel: he experienced the ultimate spiritual isolation when he died on the cross. God "made him who knew no sin," Jesus, to bear the massive weight of our sin (2 Cor. 5:21). Since God in his holiness cannot look on sin, Jesus was separated from his heavenly Father when he took on our sin.

From the depths of this isolation comes his cry, "My God, my God, why have you forsaken me?" (Matthew 27:46). Jesus' suffering love made it sure and certain that **we** would never again experience the separation from God that our sin deserves. As Scotty Smith writes in one of his daily prayers, "Your cry, 'My God, my God, why have you forsaken me?' assures us that we'll never be forsaken—**never**."[18]

As you wait, dear friend, you may feel as if you are completely alone, as if Jesus is no longer present. Remember that this is a *feeling*, not the reality; Jesus has experienced that isolation so that we may never be alone again.

PRAYER

Lord, our ever-near Father, give us your assurance this very moment that you are with us, you are in us, you are around us. By your Spirit-Comforter we pray that we may believe what is true even when we do not feel it, AMEN.

FURTHER ENCOURAGEMENT

- Read Matthew 27:45-50; Luke 23:32-34; and John 19:30.

- Read A Prayer for the Discouraged by Scotty Smith at https://www.thegospelcoalition.org/blogs/scotty-smith/a-prayer-for-the-discouraged-4/.

FOR REFLECTION

What loneliness or sense of forsakenness have you or your loved one experienced during this season?

NOTES

23

Your Helper is Here!

And I will ask the Father, and he will give you
another Helper, to be with you forever,…
JOHN 14:16, ESV

THE BURDEN OF caregiving is a heavy one; at times, we will feel crushed under the emotional, mental, and physical stress. This distress is exacerbated by the extreme isolation we sometimes experience. Missing the regular social activities of life—church, summer softball league, baby showers, weddings, and even funerals—can leave us feeling very lonely.

What if someone could send a helper, someone who would offer such good company that we would never feel alone? This helper would offer the best counsel but would never try to fix us with trite advice. This helper would even transform our suffering into glory. Guess what? This "person" actually exists—it is the third person of the Trinity, the Holy Spirit.

The Holy Spirit, John 14:16 says, is sent by God, our faithful and loving Father, at Jesus' request. The Greek word used for the Holy Spirit is *paraclete*, from the verb *parakaleo*, which means "to walk alongside." Consider the job description of the Holy Spirit as laid out for us in Scripture:

Counselor (John 14:16): The Helper is the perfect counselor and comforter. Martin Luther writes, "A counselor fills a troubled heart with joy toward God. A counselor encourages us to be happy that our sins are forgiven, death has been conquered, heaven has been opened, and God is smiling upon us."[19]

Intercessor (Romans 8:26): The Helper knows just how to pray for us, giving us the words we do not have and praying according to the will of God: "…. the Spirit helps us in our weakness. For we do not know what to pray for as we ought, but the Spirit himself intercedes for us with groanings too deep for words…the Spirit intercedes for the saints according to the will of God" (Romans 8:26-27, ESV).

Transformer (2 Corinthians 3:17-18): The Helper actually lives inside us and transforms us into the likeness of God! As Scotty Smith explains, "The Holy Spirit constantly draws attention to Jesus—nestling the gospel into our hearts and applying the finished work of Jesus to our lives."[20] As the Holy Spirit points us to the glory of God, he is actually making us more glorious! (2 Corinthians 3:18, NLT).

What a Helper we have in the Spirit! In moments when we feel painfully isolated, let us remember our Counselor, Intercessor, and Transformer, the perfect company that God has sent to us at Jesus' request!

PRAYER

Spirit of the Living God fall afresh on us. Point us to

Jesus, who points us to God, who has forgiven sins
and conquered death and restored us to new life!
With your perfect help we pray, AMEN.

FURTHER ENCOURAGEMENT

- Read John 16:5-15; Romans 8:26-27; 2 Corinthians
  3:17-18.

- Listen to "Come, O Come Thou Holy Spirit" by
  Indelible Grace at https://youtu.be/p-jJqhz1bgg.

FOR REFLECTION

In what ways has the Holy Spirit helped you during this
season? What additional help might you ask from the Holy
Spirit?

24

Unfulfilled

*And we believers also groan, even though we
have the Holy Spirit within us as a foretaste
of future glory, for we long for our bodies to be
released from sin and suffering. We, too, wait
with eager hope for the day when God will
give us our full rights as his adopted children,
including the new bodies he has promised us.*
ROMANS 8:23-24, NLT

"I'm sorry. We are unfulfilled. There is no diagnosis."

TWO DAYS AFTER our son's first brain surgery, his neurosurgeon delivered this unwelcome news. The doctor had stopped the surgery to remove the brain tumor when he discovered what he believed to be a venous malformation. Further tests were done, an angiogram and an MRI, in an attempt to discover exactly what was going on inside our son's head. The results were back, but they were inconclusive.

I loved the fact that our neurosurgeon shot straight with us: at this point, they still did not know if our son had a tumor. I *hated* the words, "unfulfilled" and "no diagnosis," and the anxiety they aroused. In this life, what we most desire, what we most yearn for, is fulfillment, a resolution to the story.

Romans 8:18-25 helps to explain the tension we feel. In the fall, creation suffered extensive damage. Weeds would grow from the once-fertile ground; sin would spread in our once-glorious beings. The whole creation, and we ourselves, now long for release from the "bondage to decay" we now endure. Romans 8:22 compares the longing for that final glorious freedom to the pangs of labor. As theologian John Stott puts it, "The indwelling Spirit gives us joy, and the coming glory gives us hope, but the interim suspense gives us pain."[21]

When the neurosurgeon first used the word *unfulfilled*, I thought it was strange, but now it makes sense. Because of his vast knowledge of the brain and extensive experience with diagnoses, he confidently expected that our hopes for a diagnosis and thus, a cure, would one day be *fulfilled*.

In the same way, we have powerful reasons to hope even as we groan for glory. We know that Christ has been raised from the dead; that knowledge gives us hope that we have been raised to new life with him (1 Corinthians 15:19-21). The Holy Spirit works in us, transforming us into new creation. This is the hope for which we were saved (Romans 8:24).

This saving hope points us toward our future hope, the day of resolution. When Christ comes again, our longings will be fulfilled. Our son's diagnosis will no longer matter, because he, and we, will be fully released from sin and suffering, in body and soul, in heart and mind. This is the hope that helps us to wait eagerly and patiently (Romans 8:24-25).

PRAYER

Oh, Lord, you hear the groanings of our hearts; you know what we long for most is you. We thank you for your Holy Spirit and your Living Word, which sustain us as we wait, AMEN.

FURTHER ENCOURAGEMENT

- Read Romans 8:18-25.

- Listen to "Our Hope Endures" by Natalie Grant at https://youtu.be/n1mu3F0dQz0.

FOR REFLECTION

What hopes do you have that are as yet "unfulfilled"? How does the future hope of Christ's return help you wait well?

25

All Will Be Well

that I may know him and the power of his
resurrection, and may share his sufferings....
PHILIPPIANS 3:10, ESV

SHORTLY AFTER OUR son's first aborted brain surgery, when it appeared that he might have to have yet another one, a friend texted me, "As you have often reminded me, 'All will be well.'" At first glance, these four small words can sound trite and insufficient, like a Band-Aid slapped on a gaping bloody wound. But when we know the context, they speak to the truest hope we have in the midst of extreme suffering.

The medieval mystic Julian of Norwich first penned the oft-quoted words, "all manner of things shall be well" in 1343 while recovering from a deathly illness. Astonishingly, as a young woman, Julian had actually prayed to experience a deathly illness so that she might better understand the suffering of Christ. After she recovered, she wrote the well-known words, explaining that although sin and sickness are inevitable in this fallen world, one day, Jesus will return, and all shall be well. [22]

Horatio Spafford is another who put the words "It is well" to his deep suffering. After his four children died in a shipwreck in 1873, he wrote the words to the comforting hymn, "It Is Well with My Soul":

> When peace like a river attendeth my way,
> When sorrows like sea-billows roll…
> Whatever my lot, Thou has taught me to say,
> "It is well, it is well with my soul." [23]

Mary Bowley Peters (1813-1856) also proclaimed that "all is well" in the midst of extreme grief. Married as a young woman to a vicar in Oxfordshire (England), she was widowed at the age of 21. In her hymn, "Through the Love of God Our Savior," also known as, "All Must Be Well," she explains the reasons for her hope:

> We expect a bright tomorrow;
>   All will be well;
> Faith can sing through days of sorrow,
>   All, all is well.
> On our Father's love relying,
>   Jesus every need supplying,
> Or in living, or in dying,
>   All must be well.[24]

Four simple words, shorthand for the fullness of hope we have in Jesus Christ. The friend who texted me those words has suffered profoundly, just as Julian, Horatio and Mary did. If those who know the "fellowship of his sufferings" can look toward the day when "all will be well," then let us join them in that hope.

PRAYER

Father God, it is only in the context of your

goodness that we can expect a bright tomorrow, that we can know all manner of things shall be well. Thank you for giving us this hope as we wait, AMEN.

FURTHER ENCOURAGEMENT

- Read Philippians 3:8-11; Romans 5:2-4; Isaiah 3:10.

- Listen to "All Must Be Well" by Indelible Grace at https://youtu.be/Y50EDNEJvTA.

FOR REFLECTION

What gives you hope that "All will be well" in this trying time?

NOTES

26

Patience and Patients

*But I received mercy for this reason, that in
me, as the foremost, Jesus Christ might display
his perfect patience as an example to those who
were to believe in him for eternal life.*
1 TIMOTHY 1:16, ESV

I WAS ACUTELY aware, even before my season of caregiving began, that I lacked the patience required for the task. In English, the word *patience* comes from a root word that means to "suffer." In the Bible, the true character of patience is exemplified by God's steadfast love and his forbearance of our sins.

Although I, like Moses, complained that I was ill-equipped for my assignment, God did not release me from the call to caregiving. God, by his Spirit, set about growing patience in me. Three essential strategies helped me remain patient when the provocation or strain of caregiving pushed me to my limit:

1. Looking at and listening to the patient's story:

Paul Miller, in his excellent book, *Love Walked among Us*, writes that Jesus' compassion was marked by his intentional way of looking at and listening to a person.[25]

99

When I grew impatient with my dad's sarcastic remarks about his new "home" in the assisted living facility, I considered what he had lost: My dad had played tennis and worked out daily at the YMCA until he was diagnosed with prostate cancer at age eight-one. He had lived on his own for over half a century. When tumors in his back and hips led us to move him to an assisted living facility, was it any wonder that he jokingly but half-seriously called it "Shawshank"?

2. Recognizing that what may feel like impatience is not always sinful:

It may simply be a normal expression of concern or a normal symptom of grief (See "Normal Grief"). If your mother won't do her PT after knee surgery (mine did!), or your husband refuses to take prescribed medicine, your frustration comes from healthy concern.

3. Running to Jesus for forgiveness when impatience led me to act unkindly.

When I lost my patience with my dad in the oncologist's waiting room and treated him unkindly (see "Forgiveness"), I needed Jesus' and my dad's forgiveness.

Dear friends, when long nights and exhausting days cause us to erupt in anger, let us flee into the compassionate arms of Jesus, whose mercy is endless and whose patience is perfect. He invites us to rest in him as completely forgiven and perfectly loved.

PRAYER

Lord God, we thank you for your unlimited supply of patience. You know we are ill-equipped for this task of perfect caregiving. We turn to the only perfect Caregiver, Jesus, for abundant mercy, AMEN.

FURTHER ENCOURAGEMENT

Read Romans 2:4; Romans 8:25; Galatians 5:22; Ephesians 4:1-3.

FOR REFLECTION

How have you struggled with patience during this season? How have you seen God's love for you when you lost patience?

27

Never Give Up

I believe that I shall look upon the goodness of
the Lord in the land of the living.
PSALM 27:13, ESV

THERE WILL BE days in the waiting room when everything seems to go wrong. You wait for hours to see the doc but then miss his rounds because you were at the pharmacy picking up a prescription; the IV isn't working, so they have to stick your beloved three more times; the pain meds don't offer much relief. The fallen world "piles on," and you feel like screaming, "I give up!"

On days like this, I called to mind a story from long ago, when our youngest son, the current patient, was just three years old.

My husband, an orthopedic surgeon, was at the hospital, where he had been for most of the previous two days, healing the broken arms of other parents' children. Our seven-year-old daughter had a stomach virus and had started the day by throwing up at various stops along her delirious route to the bathroom. The time of grace—bedtime—had finally arrived. I was tucking in our son, who, though ordinarily cheerful, was sobbing relentlessly because of a bottom rash developed in the pool.

Finally, I threw my hands in the air and yelled up to God, "I give up!" Our three-year-old piped up through his tears, delivering nine words I have never forgotten: "Mommy can't know how to give up on me!" I cringed in sorrow and shame, climbed into his little toddler bed, scooped him into my arms, and said, "No, Mommy won't give up!" About that time, our five-year-old daughter walked in, carrying a huge glass of ice water. She said, "When I don't feel good, a glass of cold water always makes me feel better."

"I give up" is the selfish cry of cynicism: things aren't going my way, they aren't getting better, and they never will. Biblical hope, tied as it is to biblical love, "never gives up" (I Cor. 13:4, The MSG), not even when the story appears to have ended tragically. God's servant David affirms this hope in Psalm 27. David believes that the Lord will make his power and presence known; he believes that the Lord's goodness will right all wrongs.

We do not give up because of our indestructible hope: Christ has died for our sins; Christ has been raised from the dead; Christ will one day come again to heal our sin-wounded souls. Hope compels us to wait courageously because we know the ending to the story, and sometimes it brings us a drink of cold water as we wait.

PRAYER:

Lord, forgive us for our impatience. Thank you for giving us your Holy Spirit, who, like a drink of cold water to our tired, thirsty souls, strengthens and encourages us for the wait. We do believe that we will see your goodness in the land of the living; help our unbelief. In Jesus' very good name we pray, AMEN.

FURTHER ENCOURAGEMENT

- Read Psalm 27.

- Listen to "Everlasting God" by Chris Tomlin at https://youtu.be/QVmaLtyOSao.

FOR REFLECTION

Have you ever felt like giving up during a long, hard wait? Has anyone brought you a "glass of cold water" as you waited? What was that experience like?

28

My Peace I Give

Peace I leave with you; my peace I give you.
I do not give to you as the world gives.
Do not let your hearts be troubled
and do not be afraid.
JOHN 14:27, NIV

A SEASON IN the waiting room brings strain and stress, doubt and dread. What we desperately need is peace. As believers, we have this peace, for Christ has left it to us as his legacy.

In Christ's farewell discourse in John 14–17, Christ prepares his disciples with the knowledge they will need to carry on his work. More than once, he assures them that he is leaving them his peace.

What is this peace that Christ leaves us? Biblical peace encompasses far more than the dictionary definition of *peace*. Our English word refers to the absence of conflict, or a state of calm. *Shalom*, the Hebrew word for peace, refers to a state of "universal flourishing, wholeness, and delight." This *shalom* gives rise to "joyful wonder" in the Creator and Savior.[26]

It is this kind of peace that Christ has left his followers, and it far surpasses the peace the world offers. Consider a few of the ways the world suggests we find peace:

107

- Conquer emotion with reason: refuse to feel pain or joy.

- Numb pain: eat, drink, work, etc. until you feel calm.

- Create security in the world: buy insurance policies, build retirement accounts, and put money in an emergency fund. (These are all good things, but they fail to bring perfect peace).

Christ's peace offers the security and rest our hearts desperately crave, especially when we are suffering. Consider a few aspects of the peace we enjoy in Christ. The peace of…

- Oneness with the Father and with one another. This is the peace Christ purchased for us on the cross; he broke down the "dividing wall of hostility" (Ephesians 2:14-16 ESV).

- Relief from the guilt of our sins, as well as relief from fear of judgment (Ephesians 2:17; Romans 5:10).

- His righteousness. The eternally right Son of the Father has made us righteous (2 Corinthians 5:21). We are now children of the King with the inheritance of princes and princesses.

- Trusting in God's goodness. Because Christ was raised from the dead, we can truly trust that God is working all things together for the good of those who love him (Romans 8:28).

- Seeing the future. As Christians, we know the end of the story. One day, when Christ returns, *shalom* will be fully and finally restored, and we will live in peace forever.

In his first post-resurrection appearance, Christ greets his disciples, "Peace be with you" (John 20:19, ESV). It is more than a greeting. It is a promise fulfilled.

PRAYER

Lord, we need your peace this very moment. Calm our hearts and fill our minds with the peace you have purchased for us. In your saving name we pray, AMEN.

FURTHER ENCOURAGEMENT

- Read John 14:27; Ephesians 2:14-17; Romans 5:10.
- Listen to "It Is Well with My Soul" by Worship Republic at https://youtu.be/GTa3p3DiEag.

FOR REFLECTION

What aspect of the peace of Christ do you most need to know right now?

29

The Peace of God

And the peace of God,
which surpasses all understanding,
will guard your hearts and
minds in Christ Jesus.
PHILIPPIANS 4:7, ESV

AFTER THE INITIAL shock of hearing that a lesion had been discovered on our son's CT-scan, I felt my body go still, my mind calm. I could only explain what I was experiencing as "the peace of God." What is this peace of God, and how in the world do we get it?

Charles Spurgeon, the great nineteenth-century preacher, illustrates the peace of God with a helpful anecdote. Once, a young boy received a treat, a sugar cube, at the nearby church. He had never tasted anything so delightful. He ran home to tell his dad about it. He tried to describe its delicious taste but could not find the words. His dad asked him many questions about the flavor, trying to understand. The boy finally said, "No, Dad, I can't explain it. Wait right here." He ran back to the church and asked for another sugar cube to share with his dad. Returning home, he gave it to his dad, who popped it in his mouth. As the sweet crystal began to melt in his mouth, his dad said, "Oh, *now* I understand."

That is what the peace of God is like. We know it when we taste it. The good news of the gospel is that all Christians experience the peace of God (See "My Peace I Give"). Our problem is that we are forgetful creatures. How can we reclaim that peace when our circumstances are difficult, when we feel anxious and despairing?

In Philippians, the apostle Paul has already instructed his readers to rejoice in the Lord, to be reasonable and kind, and to recall that the Lord is near (Philippians 4:4-5). Now he describes an additional part of the process of regaining the peace of God:

"Don't worry about anything; instead, pray about everything. Tell God what you need, and thank him for all he has done" (Philippians 4:6, NLT). As we cast our cares upon him (1 Peter 5:7), God responds with his peace; not just any peace, but a peace that surpasses all understanding.

It is a...

- **Surpassing** peace, something reason cannot grasp. It is the peace that tells us if God could raise Jesus from the dead, he can work good out of the very worst circumstances.

- **Guarding** peace, which keeps our hearts and minds secure when they head toward the quicksand of despair.

- **Trusting** peace, like a child's ease that comes from resting fully in our heavenly Father.

The peace of God is a perfect peace, a lasting peace, a blanketing peace. It is a peace that abides and drives us to wait in hope. Dear friends, let us present our requests with thanksgiving to the God who has already made peace with us and who stands ready to fill us again with his spreading shalom.

PRAYER

Lord, you have promised to keep in perfect peace all whose minds are fixed on thee. Fix our minds on you, and let our hearts rest in your peace, AMEN.

FURTHER ENCOURAGEMENT

- Read Colossians 3:15; Isaiah 26:3, 12.

- Listen to "Perfect Peace" by Laura Story at https://youtu. be/UF2iiIrWBbI.

FOR REFLECTION

How have you experienced the surpassing peace of God during your time in the waiting room?

30

The Community of Faith

Bear one another's burdens,
and so fulfill the law of Christ.
GALATIANS 6:2, ESV

"MY FEELINGS ARE tired." These wise words were first spoken by a three-year-old, whose mother passed them on to me. They aptly describe the impact a health crisis can have on patients and loved ones.

On several occasions during his health crisis, our son expressed concern about his struggle to pray and read his Bible. As I reminded him, it is normal during severe loss to experience spiritual weariness. I also encouraged him to allow the community of faith, the church universal, to carry him during this season.

In his stellar work on grief, *A Grace Disguised*, Dr. Jerry Sittser, who lost his mother, wife, and daughter in a car accident, writes about how the community of faith carried him. I emailed him to ask more about this aspect of grief, and he graciously responded:

> "The church is a community. Sometimes some
> members of that community, even through time

and space, carry others, because we do not have the capacity to function the same way. I remember very vividly my inability to sing and pray, especially sing, in the months and, really, years after the accident. I decided to let the church sing and pray for me, not only the church here and now but the church everywhere and, well, 'everywhen.' I do the same for others now. I sing for them; I pray for them."[27]

Reading Dr. Sittser's words, I remembered how my husband used to occasionally hoist one of our young children onto his shoulders for a free ride. From high above, they could see around the crowd at a busy festival, as their tired little legs could rest during a long walk. In the same way, the church is called to bear one another's burdens, to "encourage the faint-hearted and help the weak" (1 Thessalonians 5:14, ESV). Love bears all things, believes all things, hopes all things and endures all things (1 Corinthians 13:7, ESV). The church likewise

- **Bears** the weight of our weary souls.

- **Believes** God's goodness for us when we struggle with doubt.

- **Hopes** for us when we are weary of waiting for redemption.

- **Endures** hardship with us as we suffer.

When our feelings are tired, we need do only one thing—receive the help offered. When my husband carried our children on his shoulders, they rode happily. They did not complain that he was carrying too heavy a burden. They simply enjoyed their new view and the rest for their legs. Jesus, by his grace, has given us an entire community to sustain us when we are weak: the church universal. Let us thank God for this strong transport and enjoy the ride. One day, soon enough, we will be called and strengthened to lift the weak to our shoulders for a respite.

PRAYER

God, we thank you for giving us the church created by Jesus Christ. Help us to humble ourselves to receive the faith, hope, and love your community has to offer us in our weak and weary state. In Jesus' loving name we pray, AMEN.

FURTHER ENCOURAGEMENT

- Read 1 Thessalonians 5:14; 1 Corinthians 13:7; Hebrews 10:24-25.

- Watch "Adversity as Spiritual Formation" (video) by Dr. Gerald Sittser at https://cct.biola.edu/adversity-spiritual-formation/

FOR REFLECTION

How has the community of faith supported you during this season? Or, if you have not felt that support, how can you reach out to the community of faith to ask for support?

NOTES

31

When You Are Weak

For when I am weak, then I am strong.
2 CORINTHIANS 12:10, ESV

THROUGHOUT MY LIFE, my father always praised my "strength"; his awe for this strength only grew as he observed how I walked through our son's health crisis. I always tried to direct what I felt was his misplaced praise to the true source of my strength: Jesus. The following is an excerpt of a texting conversation we once had about this subject:

> **My dad:** *You are incredibly strong in a day after day exceedingly trying time…no one knows how you do it….*
>
> **Me:** *Jesus!*
>
> **My dad:** *"My strength and my Redeemer?"*
>
> **Me:** *Oh yes!*

I often struggled under my dad's praise of my strength as if it were a man's heavy leather jacket placed on the shoulders of a small child. Why? Because I've learned that it is dangerous to put my faith in my own strength. Because I know that I am frequently tempted to rely on myself alone; I am easily seduced by self-reliance.

In 2 Corinthians 12:7-10, Paul explains God's upside-down way of thinking about strength and weakness. Paul had a "thorn in the flesh" which scholars across the ages have failed to identify. He pleaded with God to remove it, but God said "no," explaining, "My grace is sufficient for you, for my power is made perfect in weakness" (v.9). Paul shares this paradox through his writing: in our weakness, we turn to Christ, who by his submission to weakness, gained power over sin and death.

As you linger in the waiting room, dear friends, I imagine you will reckon with, as I have, the wide range and profound depth of your weaknesses. Perhaps...

- Your temper is short with patient and medical staff.

- Your faith in the Lord is fragile, tossing with every wave of medical report.

- Your competence, which has served you well in your job, has no power to shorten your wait time in seeing the doctor or receiving diagnostic results.

- Your physical stamina, which got you through a half-marathon last year, is waning, and all you want to do is sleep for a very long time in your own bed.

Paul Tripp explains that our weakness is actually very good news:

> God chooses for you to be weak to protect you from you and to cause you to value the strength which only he can give.... these weaknesses are tools of his zealous and amazing grace.... They keep you from

thinking that you are capable of what you're not. They remind you that you are needy and were created to be dependent on One greater than you. They cause you to do what all of us in some way resist doing—humbly run to God for the help that only he can give.[28]

PRAYER

Lord, forgive us for trying to live life in the waiting room in our own strength. Help us to rest in you, our Strength and our Redeemer, AMEN.

FURTHER ENCOURAGEMENT

- Read 2 Corinthians 12:7-10; Philippians 2:5-11.
- Listen to "The Weight of the World" by Rain for Roots at https://youtu.be/mvTZpYTUNtI

FOR REFLECTION

What weaknesses have you struggled with during this season? How might these weaknesses be a good thing?

32

Self-Care: Your Body Is a Temple

...for you were bought with a price.
So glorify God in your body.
1 CORINTHIANS 6:20, ESV

STRANDS OF HAIR remained on my hand after I rubbed the shampoo into my head. Moments later, while brushing my hair, more strands came out. I stopped and took a good look at myself in the mirror for the first time in days. Dark trenches had dug in deep beneath my bleary eyes. My face looked pale and gray. The reality was clear: my body was losing the war to stress.

It is very tempting to be care-*less* of our own physical needs as we wait, but the God who cherishes us asks us to care well for our own bodies even as we care for others.

When our son was recovering and my father's health was deteriorating rapidly, I tended to think that I was the **only one** who could care well for them. Author Amie Patrick's words about self-care resonate: "I avoided self-care because it looked dangerously close to self-indulgence. But avoiding self-care actually fed my sinful appetite to live self-sufficiently and to seek fulfillment in my own abilities…. God taught me that self-denial for me meant stopping to rest."[29]

I, like Amie, needed to stop to rest, to hear Jesus' call, "Come to me, all you who are weary and carry heavy burdens, and I will give you rest" (Matthew 11:28, NLT). But how can we rest when our loved ones have so many needs?

- Look to Jesus who took breaks for solitude, prayer, rest, and feasting. Certainly, Jesus cared for numerous people who had desperate needs, and yet at times he intentionally rested from those needs, seeking time with his heavenly Father and giving respite to his body. Following his example, we can take a walk outside of the hospital or house, enjoying some fresh air and asking God for strength to sustain us through another day.

- Look to the church. Christ's church is designed to share burdens. The fact is, people want to *do* something; therefore, we are actually blessing another by asking them to come sit with our loved one or accepting offers of meals, lawn-mowing or dog-sitting.

- Look to God as provider. Remember that the God who became flesh and blood knows our every physical need. He does indeed provide for our bodies when we are in a season of crisis, but he also gives us skilled physicians and wise counselors to advise us on how to get enough sleep in times of stress or how to address blood pressure that has sky-rocketed.

It is hard, dear friend, but not impossible, to be kind to your own body even as you care lovingly for another's. Hear God's call to come to him and rest.

PRAYER

Dear Father, you knit us together, designed our very bodies for glory. Help us remember, even as we suffer the effects of stress, how very well you care for us. Teach us to care well for ourselves by your grace and provision. In Jesus' rest-giving name we pray, AMEN.

FURTHER ENCOURAGEMENT

Read Matthew 11:28-30; Luke 5:16; John 2:1; 1 Corinthians 6:20; Galatians 6:2.

FOR REFLECTION

What effects of stress do you observe in yourself? What actions of self-care have been helpful to you?

33

Searching for Signs of Redemption

*So these stones shall be to the people
of Israel a memorial forever.*
JOSHUA 4:7, ESV

IN MANY HOSPITALS and doctors' offices, the lovely efforts of interior designers have brought beauty to the dreary setting. Still, when we are daily faced with the pallor of our loved one, when we look around at the steely surfaces and hard beige plastic of medical equipment, we can feel oppressed by our surroundings. It is crucial, then, that we look for signs of redemption everywhere.

Joshua 4 tells the story of the Israelites crossing the Jordan River into the Promised Land. The Lord has miraculously dried up the powerful river. He instructs Joshua to tell his people to gather stones from the dried riverbed and make a memorial out of them (Joshua 4:1-3). Joshua tells the people, "In the future your children will ask you, 'What do these stones mean?' Then you can tell them, 'They remind us that the Jordan River stopped flowing when the Ark of the Lord's Covenant went across.' These stones will stand as a memorial among the people of Israel forever" (Joshua 4:6-7, NLT).

This story reminds us to seek signs of redemption anywhere

and everywhere. God reveals himself not only through Scripture but also through his creation. If we look, we will find messages from God etched into the very universe we inhabit. As Psalm 19:1 explains:

"The heavens declare the glory of God,
and the sky above proclaims his handiwork"
(ESV).

Similarly, the apostle Paul asserts, "For what can be known about God is plain to them, because God has shown it to them" (Romans 1:19, ESV). In other words, we will see God's glory if we are looking for it. But God also has brought his unique message of love to me through heart shapes found in nature and sunflowers sighted in unexpected places. In my mental collection of love letters from God, you might find a heart-shaped stone, cloud, or leaf; bubble-gum stamped in the sidewalk in the shape of a heart; or a lone sunflower growing on the side of the expressway. Each of these reminds me that in addition to sending us a love letter in his Holy Word, God continues to send messages of redemption in our everyday lives by providing glimpses of beauty that delight our hearts..

Frederick Buechner encourages us to have the faith "to wait, to watch, to listen, for the incredible presence of God here in the world among us."[30] Look carefully today, dear friend, and see what signs of redemption our gracious God has sent to you.

PRAYER

Lord, give us the faith to see you at work even in the "stuff and nonsense" of our days. Help us to see the signs of restoration work you have painted in

Scripture and in your world, AMEN.

- Read Psalm 19:1-6; Isaiah 61:1-3.

- Listen to "There You Are" by Carolyn Arends at https://www.youtube.com/watch?v=lVHCWW-aCNs

FOR REFLECTION

What signs of beauty or redemption have you seen along this journey? How have these signs reminded you of God's nearness to you?

NOTES

34

When God Said "No"

> *'Father, if you are willing,*
> *remove this cup from me.*
> *Nevertheless, not my will,*
> *but yours, be done.'*
> LUKE 22:42, ESV

SEVENTEEN DAYS AFTER our son's second surgery, his wound became infected. He would have to undergo a third surgery to wash out the wound. The neurosurgeon forewarned me that if the bone flap (part of the skull they had removed to access his brain) was infected, they would need to remove it, then return in six months to insert a synthetic one. During the surgery, I sat alone in the waiting room, pleading with God, "Lord, please don't let that bone be infected. Please don't let our son have to have a fourth surgery." Two hours later, I learned that God had said *no.*

What do we do during this strenuous waiting season when God answers *no* to specific and heartfelt prayers? There is really only one thing to do: turn to Jesus. Because of one of the most emphatic *no*'s ever delivered, Jesus was sent to the cross. Let's visit Jesus in the Garden of Gethsemane where he agonizes in prayer.

Jesus has become sorrowful and troubled (Matthew 26:37) as he considers the torment he faces. He instructs his disciples to wait and pray while he goes farther into the garden, falls on his face and pleads with God. He asks God to "remove the cup." To drink the cup is to bear God's wrath for the sake of our sins, to be separated from God, his beloved Father. Luke describes God's response to Jesus' first prayer: "And there appeared to him an angel from heaven, strengthening him" (Luke 22:43, ESV). God told him neither *yes* nor *no* but sent an angel to strengthen him.

Even with the angels' strengthening, Jesus remains in agony, sweating drops of blood (Luke 22:44). He prays "more earnestly," affirming his submission to God's will: "My Father, if this cannot pass unless I drink it, your will be done" (Matthew 26:42, ESV). Jesus leaves the place, returns to his disciples, finds them sleeping, then goes back and prays a third time, "saying the same words again" (Matthew 26:44, ESV).

God said *no* to Jesus' request that the cup pass from him. It is this *no* that bought us the *yes* of God forever. Jesus "endured the cross, despising the shame, for the joy set before him" (Hebrews 12:2, ESV). Jesus' joy was to bring us to his Father, to hear his Father say *yes* to adopting us as his children.

Now we have confidence that our Father loves to hear our requests because we are "heirs according to the promise" (Galatians 3:29, ESV). We find peace and hope, even in the answer of *no* because we know that our good, good Father gives the best gifts to his children (Luke 11:11).

PRAYER

Gracious heavenly Father, thank you for hearing and answering our prayers. Help us to have peace and hope, even when your answer is *no.* In Jesus' praying name we ask, AMEN.

FURTHER ENCOURAGEMENT

- Read Luke 22:39-46; Matthew 26:36-46.

- Listen to "Thy Will Be Done" by Indelible Grace at https://indeliblegrace.bandcamp.com/track/ thy-will-be-done.

FOR REFLECTION

What prayers has God said "no" to during this season? Write or say a prayer asking him to speak comfort into your disappointment.

35

When You Mistake Jesus for a Ghost

*But when the disciples saw him walking on the
sea, they were terrified, and said, 'It is a ghost!'
and they cried out in fear.*
MATTHEW 14:26, ESV

AT TIMES DURING a health crisis, fear and weariness may lead
you to believe you are seeing a ghost—that is, something that
seems harmful. You may eventually discover that this initially
terrifying apparition is in fact Jesus, coming to save you in the
storm.

Once, after a long night on a stormy sea, the disciples mistook Jesus for a ghost (Matthew 14:22-33). Earlier that day,
the disciples watched astounded as Jesus miraculously transformed two fish and five loaves into a feast for well over five
thousand people. As soon as the feast ended, Jesus sent his
disciples to cross the sea of Galilee in their boat, and he headed
up the mountain to pray.

Out on the sea, a fierce storm arises, so fierce that it bul-
lies the disciples even though many are seasoned fishermen.
According to the accounts in John and Mark, the disciples
have been rowing for around ten hours and have only traveled
about three miles. They are weary and frightened.

When the disciples see a dim figure walking toward them through the spraying sea and lashing rain, they imagine it to be a ghost. On the one hand, we can understand how their fear and exhaustion leads them to this conclusion. On the other hand, have they so quickly forgotten that Jesus had miraculously whipped up a delicious dinner for five thousand out of a couple of fish and some barley loaves?

I know how they felt. On the day of our son's third surgery, the one to wash out the infected wound, I was weary and frightened. When the surgeon told me the results—the bone flap had been infected; he had removed a cell-phone-sized section of the skull—I crumpled in my chair. I had seen a ghost: I envisioned as terrible apparitions all of the things to come: six weeks of IV antibiotics, yet another surgery in six months to replace the removed skull piece. The doctor reassured me, "Elizabeth, he's going to do great!" He knew that what he had found was hopeful news: the bone was infected, but the brain itself was not.

When I mistook Jesus for a ghost, I had lost sight of the Jesus who fed large crowds with inadequate resources. In that moment, I did not recognize the Jesus who brings hope and calm in the midst of a maelstrom.

Dear friends, if you think you are seeing a ghost, hear the words Jesus spoke to his disciples that night on the stormy sea, "Take heart; it is I. Do not be afraid" (Matthew 14:27, ESV).

PRAYER

Precious Lord Jesus, you are so very kind to your disciples, calling out to us in our fearful imaginings. We praise you as the Lord who rules over all creation, feeding us with your hope, calming us with your peace. In your saving name we pray, AMEN.

FURTHER ENCOURAGEMENT

Read Matthew 14:22-33.

FOR REFLECTION

What experiences do you have of mistaking Jesus for a ghost along this journey? Have you seen things you thought were harmful that in fact turned out for good?

NOTES

36

Steadfast

The steadfast love of the Lord never ceases; His
mercies never come to an end.
LAMENTATIONS 3:22, ESV

IN THE TOPSY-TURVY waiting room days, we need to remember that the Lord's love is steadfast, that it never ceases, and that his mercies never come to an end. Perhaps you are like me, and you did not realize that those verses of comfort and reassurance come smack in the middle of one of the most harrowing expressions of sorrow in the entire Bible, the book of Lamentations. Realizing this assertion about God's firm, fixed love arises during a season of desperation gives us hope, even on the darkest days.

Lamentations, authored perhaps by the prophet Jeremiah, describes in graphic detail the devastation following the fall of Jerusalem to Babylon. It is *not* bedtime reading, given its gut-wrenching descriptions of children and mothers starving in the streets, and mothers actually eating "the fruit of their womb" (Lamentations 2:19-20, ESV). The destruction of Jerusalem was a direct result of the Israelites' failure to obey and worship God. The author's lament rises to the Lord, who, he points out, "fulfilled the promises of disaster he made long ago" by sending Babylon to destroy God's holy city. The author cries out to the Lord for mercy, asking, "Should you treat your own people this way?" (Lam. 2:20, NLT). And then, right in the middle of his cry, the author seems to suddenly remember—there *is* cause for hope:

> But this I call to mind,
> And therefore I have hope:
> The steadfast love of the Lord never ceases;
> His mercies never come to an end (Lam. 3:22, ESV).

The steadfast love of the Lord is a balm to apply to all kinds of suffering:

- When we are like "the one who has seen the afflictions that come from the rod of the Lord's anger" (Lam. 3:1, NLT), "The steadfast love of the Lord never ceases."

- When we feel that "peace has been stripped away" (Lam. 3:17, NLT), "The steadfast love of the Lord never ceases."

- When we think we will "never forget this awful time" (Lam. 3:20, NLT), "The steadfast love of the Lord never ceases."

What the author knows with certainty, is that the Lord's steadfast love meets us in our suffering—steadfastly. Firmly. Fixedly. Without moving. Without turning away. It is the Lord's steadfast love that sent Jesus to earth as a man and sent Jesus to the cross to die for our sins. It is the Lord's steadfast love that raised Jesus from the dead and raises us to new life in Christ. It is the Lord's steadfast love that will send Jesus back one day to take his people home; this same steadfast love will wipe away all tears in that day.

PRAYER

Lord, surely it is good that we should "wait quietly for the salvation of the Lord" (Lam. 3:25, ESV). We cry out in our suffering, looking to be stilled by your certain response of comforting love. In Jesus' saving name we pray, AMEN.

FURTHER ENCOURAGEMENT

- Read Lamentations 3:1-33.
- Listen to "Steadfast" by Sandra McCracken at https://youtu.be/SlsFC6RzUNk.

FOR REFLECTION

In what way have you seen the steadfast love of the Lord in the waiting room? What brings you hope today?

NOTES

37

Jesus Has His Eyes on You

But when he saw the wind, he was afraid,
and beginning to sink he cried out,
'Lord, save me.' Jesus immediately reached
out his hand and took hold of him...
MATTHEW 14:30-31, ESV

AFTER OUR SON'S third surgery, we were tasked with infusing him with IV antibiotics three times daily. Lacking any medical training, I felt very anxious about my nursing duties and prayed frequently for help. It was challenging, but I was toddling along, taking baby steps on the tumultuous sea.

Around this same time, my dad's condition worsened, and we began scurrying to get him appropriate pain management and care. As the wind kicked up and waves splashed my face, I started to sink under the weight of worry. To make matters worse, I chastised myself for my lack of faith.

Then, while preparing a Bible study about Jesus and Peter walking on the water (Matthew 14:28-32), I read Daniel Doriani's commentary on the passage. He notes that people often mistakenly read the passage as a morality tale about Peter: either he is praised as a bold risk-taker for his faith in stepping into the stormy sea, or he is chided for his failure of faith when he begins to sink. While Peter does demonstrate both courageous faith and lack thereof, Doriani reminds us that the story, like the whole Bible, points to Jesus: "The moral of the story is not therefore that Peter is flawed because he took his eyes off Jesus. The lesson is that Peter's failure does not matter *because Jesus did not take his eyes off Peter.*"[31]

The story's primary focus is Jesus, not Peter. It is about the Jesus who calls Peter to come to him (Matthew 14:29), the Jesus who empowers him to step out of the boat into the raging sea. It is about the Jesus whose eyes never leave Peter, even when Peter's eyes leave Jesus. It is about the Jesus who *immediately* reaches out his hand and takes hold of Peter (Matthew 14:31), pulling him out of the waves, saving him when he calls out. And yes, it is about the Jesus who gently rebukes Peter, calling him a "little-faith," asking him why he doubted (Matthew 14:31).

We are all "little-faith's." But Jesus is gentle with Peter, and he is gentle with us. When we sink in fear as Peter did, let's call out to Jesus as Peter did. The one who has his eyes firmly fixed on us will grip us tightly, lifting us up and steadying us as we return to safe harbor. This is the hope of the gospel and the hope of a growing faith.

PRAYER

Saving Lord Jesus, you know our hearts inside and out. You know when we trust in your power, and you know when we take our eyes off you and begin to sink in seas of doubt. We are so grateful you never take your eyes off us, and we are astonished that you always love to look at us. In your ever-faithful name we pray, AMEN.

Read Matthew 14:22-33.

FOR REFLECTION

In what ways have you been like Peter during your season in the waiting room, either fully focused on Jesus, or taking your eyes off of Jesus?

NOTES

38

The Kindness of Strangers

*'For I was hungry and you gave me food, I was
thirsty and you gave me drink, I was a stranger
and you welcomed me, I was naked and you
clothed me, I was sick and you visited me, I
was in prison and you came to me.'*
MATTHEW 25:35-36, ESV

WHEN OUR LOVED ones are in health crisis, we often find ourselves far away from home and utterly dependent on the kindness of strangers. We lived four hours away from the hospital where our son had four surgeries. Many friends and friends of friends offered us room in their home, but we usually stayed in the hotel adjoining the hospital so we could get back for quick naps and food from our "refrigerator," a stocked cooler.

One day, though, when our son was unexpectedly admitted for an extended stay because of infection, I returned to our hotel to discover there was no more "room in the inn" for me. I had only booked the room for two nights, and the hotel was overbooked the rest of the week for a conference. I was—temporarily—homeless. Thankfully, the kind clerk at my current hotel-home quickly arranged for me to stay at a sister-hotel just two blocks away at a highly discounted rate.

In this distressing situation and many others like it, the Lord met me with the kindness of strangers.

It is in the nature of a Christian to be kind to strangers. Jesus, in talking about the end times, makes the surprising point that in caring for the needy, we are caring for him. In Matthew 25, Jesus says that one day, he will welcome those who fed, clothed, sheltered, and visited him (Matthew 25:35-36). The "righteous ones," not realizing they have done these things for Jesus, will question him, and he will assure them, "…when you did it to the least of these my brothers and sisters, you were doing it to me" (Matthew 25:40, NLT). As I read this passage, I considered the implications of our waiting room experience:

- Kind strangers have fed us bounteous meals during this season. In doing so, they have fed Jesus. At the same time, they have pointed us to the feast we will one day enjoy with the King of the new heavens and the new earth.

- Kind strangers have offered us a home when we were homeless. In doing so, they have housed Jesus even as they have pointed us to Jesus' heavenly mansion.

- Kind strangers have visited our son when he was sick. They have cared for Jesus even as they point us to the Christ who visited this world in the flesh and will one day take us home.

The kindness shown by strangers leads us to wait well for the Day Jesus will return to welcome us into his kingdom.

PRAYER

Dear Jesus, may we all know and appreciate the extraordinary kindness of strangers during this odd season. We look forward to the day when you will welcome them, and us, to your celebration feast. In your kind name we pray, AMEN.

FURTHER ENCOURAGEMENT

Read Matthew 25:31-46; Hebrews 13:2.

FOR REFLECTION

In what ways have you experienced the kindness of strangers during this season? What kindness have you offered to strangers?

39

The Embrace of the Father

And he arose and came to his father.
But while he was still a long way off,
his father saw him and felt compassion,
and ran and embraced him and kissed him.
LUKE 15:20, ESV

IT WAS LATE afternoon on the day before my dad's memorial service. Our twenty-six-year-old daughter was at the kitchen table studying, and our twenty-two-year-old son was working on his computer. I was puttering around the kitchen, waiting on my brother to arrive. My husband, brother, and I were headed to the beach to toss my dad's ashes in the Gulf of Mexico.

Suddenly, I stopped cleaning the counter, turned to my daughter and son and voiced my frustration, "I don't know how to do this! I've never scattered ashes before…. I don't have any experience!" My daughter stood, came to me and wrapped her arms around me, gathering me in and holding me close. It is a hug I will never forget. It felt like the embrace of our heavenly Father.

The parable Jesus told in Luke 15:11-32, often entitled the "Prodigal Son," is better understood when we focus on the embracing father. The story begins with a selfish son committing a grave Ancient Near Eastern offense in demanding his inheritance from his father. In that culture, to ask for your inheritance early was like saying, "I wish you were dead." The young son then runs off to a distant land and spends everything on "reckless living" (Luke 15:13, ESV). A famine arises in the country, and the son realizes his desperation when he finds himself longing to eat the food of the pigs he is paid to feed. He schemes up a plan: he will return home and ask his father if he can work as a hired hand. At this point in the story, we see the wild prodigality of the father (*prodigal* actually means "characterized by profuse or wasteful expenditure"[32]).

In this parable, Jesus shows us what the embrace of God, our heavenly Father, is like. It is…

- The embrace of a *waiting* father who longs for the return of his wandering and squandering children.

- The embrace of a *pursuing* father who does something unthinkable in his culture by picking up his robes and running to greet his returning son.

- The embrace of a *celebrating* father who welcomes the wayward child home with a kiss, a robe, and a feast.

- The embrace of an *inviting* father who leaves the party, seeking out the elder child who is too stuck in his own righteousness to celebrate.

Finally, the parable draws attention to the seemingly reckless sacrifice of our heavenly Father, who "did not spare his own Son but gave him up for us all" (Romans 8:32, ESV). Dear friend, during this most trying season, may you know the embrace of this Father who "graciously give(s) us all things" (Romans 8:32, ESV).

PRAYER

Oh, prodigal Father, thank you for welcoming me to the feast, wayward and proud child that I am. Help me to know your embrace and share it with others. In Jesus' prodigal name we pray, AMEN.

FURTHER ENCOURAGEMENT

- Read Luke 15:11-31.

- Listen to "Communion Hymn" by Stuart Townend at https://youtu.be/S1rQy1TrgXI

FOR REFLECTION

How have you experienced the embrace of the heavenly Father during this season?

40

The Wrong Question

But some of them said, 'Could not
he who opened the eyes of the blind man
also have kept this man from dying?'
JOHN 11:37, ESV

DURING A HEALTH CRISIS, we often ask the wrong question of Jesus. We know he has the power to heal, so, like Lazarus' friends, we ask why he hasn't healed yet. Jesus seems to want us to ask him a different question: "Who are you?" This question is the one Jesus answers in the story of Lazarus' illness.

Lazarus is ill, and his sisters Mary and Martha send for Jesus. Jesus, hearing the news, tells his disciples, "This illness does not lead to death. It is for the glory of God, that the Son of Man might be glorified through it" (John 11:4, ESV). Immediately, Jesus draws the focus away from the physical healing of man to the glorification of God.

Next, we are told two facts that are apparently connected: Jesus loved the sisters and Lazarus, **"so"** he waited two days before going to them (John 11:5-6). At first, we are puzzled—if Jesus loved Lazarus, why did he not hurry to heal him? As we return to the story, we realize Jesus has a greater purpose in his love.

By the time Jesus arrives, Lazarus is dead. Martha expresses first her disappointment, then her remarkable faith. First, she tells Jesus that Lazarus would not have died if he had been there. Then she affirms that she knows God will give Jesus whatever he asks. (John 11:21-22, ESV). Martha has strong faith, but she is still focusing primarily on the healing of Lazarus.

As Jesus responds to Martha, he gently turns her focus toward what he really wants her to see: "I am the resurrection and the life. Whoever believes in me, though he die, yet shall he live, and everyone who lives and believes in me shall never die" (John 11:25-26, ESV). He follows this profound revelation with the crucial question, "Do you believe this?" (John 11:26, ESV).

This was the question that I longed for my father to answer affirmatively when he was diagnosed with prostate cancer. For two years after his diagnosis, he could not or would not share that answer with me.

Something happened with my dad, though, when our son had to undergo three brain surgeries in a five-week period. After we finally received the news that the mass removed from our son's brain was not a cancerous tumor, my dad texted me, "To God be the glory." Ten days later, my dad died. When I went to see him an hour after his death, his body was at rest, his face peaceful. He looked like a man who believed in Jesus, the resurrection and the life.

So often I had asked Jesus, "Why is our son having to suffer so much?" Now I can hear Jesus' answer in his words to his disciples: "This happened so that the Son of God may be glorified" (John 11:4, ESV).

PRAYER

Lord God, forgive us for being more concerned with the "why" than the "who." Help us to see **you,** working for your glory and our good in this current story. May we know and believe in the power of your resurrection, AMEN.

FURTHER ENCOURAGEMENT

Read John 11:1-37.

FOR REFLECTION

Have you focused more on the "why" than the "who" during this health crisis? What do you think Jesus might want you to see?

NOTES

Jesus Wept

Jesus wept.
JOHN 11:35, ESV

DO YOU FEEL LIKE CRYING? Perhaps your loved one has just been told they will have to have yet another needle stuck in them. Or maybe it's the lab report—you had hoped all signs of infection would be gone, but they're not. You are weary of all the loss and pain, and you begin to weep.

In Western culture, we often miss the value of mourning, but the Bible says, "Blessed are those who mourn, for they shall be comforted" (Matthew 5:4, ESV). All of God's people mourn, including Jesus. To better understand why mourning is so important, let's return to the scene in Bethany, where Lazarus has died.

Jesus has met Martha's sorrow with the life-changing revelation that he is the resurrection and the life. Now Mary comes to him, falling at his feet, weeping. John 11:33 picks up the story: "When Jesus saw her weeping, and the Jews who had come with her also weeping, he was deeply moved in his spirit and greatly troubled." Jesus is taken to the tomb, where John tells us, "Jesus wept" (John 11:35, ESV). What was it that caused Jesus to be so "deeply moved" and "greatly troubled" that he wept?

- Jesus wept because his dear friends and their community wept. Although Jesus knew that Lazarus' death would end in resurrection, bringing glory to God, he felt the pain of those who suffered Lazarus' loss. As you weep, dear friend, take comfort in Jesus, the "sympathetic priest" who feels the agony of those he loves (Hebrews 4:15).

- Jesus wept because he saw the brutal effects of sin: "His holy tears are those of the Creator grieving over the forfeiture of beauty through the intrusion of sin and death."[33] As you weep, dear friend, know that Jesus also grieved over the brokenness you are experiencing.

- Jesus wept because he knew that his own death was imminent. He dreaded being separated from God. Jesus knew that on the cross, all of God's wrath for our sins would be poured out on him. As he took on our sins, he would be separated from his Father, with whom he had been united since before time began. As you weep, dear friend, weep for gratitude that Jesus made a way for all broken things, including our sin, to be restored.

Considering the depth of Jesus' mourning, perhaps we in Western culture weep too rarely, not too often. Let us mourn now, dear friends, for "Weeping may tarry for the night, but joy comes with the morning" (Psalm 30:5).

PRAYER

Lord Jesus, thank you for weeping real tears that we might know the agony you suffered on our behalf.

Help us to weep freely over the brokenness we see around us, and comfort us with the hope of your joy and your new morning mercies. In your weeping name we pray, AMEN.

FURTHER ENCOURAGEMENT

- Read John 11:17-53.

- Listen to "Come to Jesus" by Chris Rice at https://youtu.be/ZyaA_ttbI8E

FOR REFLECTION

What makes you want to weep during this season? Do you have a sense that God joins you in your sorrow?

42

Worth Waiting For

*I will tell of the Lord's unfailing love. I will
praise the Lord for all he has done. I will
rejoice in his great goodness to Israel, which he
has granted according to his mercy and love.*
ISAIAH 63:7, NLT

AFTER OUR SON'S second brain surgery, a small piece of his
skull had become infected, and the neurosurgeon had removed
it. Six months later, they would implant a synthetic skull piece
to replace the one removed. We were all eager for our son to
have this fourth, and hopefully, final surgery.

The day finally arrived for this surgery. When we arrived
at pre-op at the appointed time, ten a.m., there was a delay;
we were asked to remain in the surgical waiting area. Finally,
around noon, our son was taken to pre-op. Forty-five minutes
later, my husband and I were invited back to wait with him.
An hour went by, then two. We were told that the neurosurgeon was involved in a very complex surgery; we'd have to
wait a while longer. As the wait was extended, my restlessness
increased, but my husband and our son remained fairly calm.
Finally, at 6 p.m., eight hours after he had been told to report,
our son was taken back to surgery. Less than two hours later,

the surgery was over, and all was well.

Amy Carmichael, missionary to India, puts words to how I felt in that "longest wait:"

> ...sometimes we are tempted to discouragement. So often we have believed that what we asked was about to be given, and then have been disappointed. *But delays are for the trial of faith, not for its discouragement.*" [emphasis added][34]

In the delay, my faith had indeed been tried. I held my tongue, because I did not want to infect our son with my anxiety, but internally, I was fantasizing about running down the hall of pre-op, screaming, "We can't take this anymore!" I later asked our son, "How did you stand that long wait?" He answered very simply, "I knew they were going to come get me eventually."

In order to wait well, we must know that the Lord is "going to come get us eventually." As Isaiah 63:7-9 reminds us, we have every reason to believe in the Lord's unfailing love. Despite Israel's repeated disobedience, the Lord has shown them "great goodness," "which he has granted according to his mercy and love" (Isaiah 63:7, NLT). As Isaiah also reminds us, "In all their suffering, he also suffered, and he personally rescued them...." (Isaiah 63:9, NLT).

Indeed, we have every reason to trust. God did not delay in sending Jesus to rescue us from the suffering of our sin. And, though it may seem like a long wait, God does not delay in sending Jesus back for us. When Jesus arrives, we will affirm, as Amy Carmichael so eloquently writes, "'Lord, this was worth waiting for.'"[35]

PRAYER

Lord, in our longest waits, help us to remember your unfailing love and abundant mercy. May we never forget that you are coming back for us and that the sweet reunion will be worth the wait, AMEN.

FURTHER ENCOURAGEMENT

- Read Isaiah 63:7-9; Isaiah 65:17-25.

- Listen to "It's Hard to Wait" by Flo Paris at https://youtu.be/HbMsm328cu8

FOR REFLECTION

What delays have you experienced during this journey? What helps you to wait well?

NOTES

43

The Gentleness of Jesus

Let your gentleness be evident to all.
PHILIPPIANS 4:5A, NIV

IT IS TEMPTING for patients to indulge in a sense of entitlement, a mindset that says, "I am suffering; I deserve to get what I want when I want it." Because this me-first attitude is so common and understandable, when a patient exhibits gentleness, it is particularly compelling.

My dad displayed such a gentleness throughout his season in the waiting room. When we arrived at the cancer center, he would shake the parking attendant's hand and ask how his day was going. As he checked in, he exchanged pleasantries with the clerk, and when the nurse arrived to take him back, he asked her thoughtful questions about her family. Although he had every reason to be grumpy, he went out of his way to be gentle and kind.

The gentleness Paul describes in Philippians 4:5 is a quality displayed by a person who has power and yet chooses to humble herself and submit to others. It is the gentleness of Jesus. Philippians 2:6-7 describes Jesus' gentleness: "Though he was God, he did not think of equality with God as something to cling to. Instead, he gave up his divine privileges; he took the humble position of a slave and was born as a human being" (NLT). Christ was gentle in the fullest sense of the word.

We observe this gentleness in Jesus as he hangs on the cross, dying for our sins. Though he is in agony, having been beaten nearly to death even before he was nailed to the cross, he hears the cries of the repentant thief. It's a small, tiny slice of a story, and it goes like this:

There are three crosses on which hang two thieves and Jesus. One thief, an "entitled" thief, makes demands of Jesus, ordering him to save them all. The second thief, a humbled, repentant thief, rebukes the first thief, pointing out that **they** deserve their punishment, whereas Christ is not guilty. The second thief then appeals to Jesus' mercy, "Jesus, remember me when you come into your kingdom" (Luke 23: 42, ESV).

Now we see the true gentleness of Jesus, just moments before his death, pronouncing these words, "Truly I say to you, today you will be with me in Paradise" (Luke 23:43, ESV). We can imagine him speaking them so very tenderly, and yet with such great authority. Jesus offers no trite words of false reassurance to the unrepentant thief. Moments later, Luke tells us, Jesus "breathed his last" (Luke 23:46, ESV).

Though he deserved to be served, Christ our Lord turned the tables, serving the lost, sick, imprisoned, and impoverished. In dying for the thief's sins and for ours, our Lord has empowered us to live a gentleness that is evident to all, even in this harsh season of waiting.

PRAYER

Lord, strengthen us, by your Spirit, to follow you in a life of service. May everyone we meet encounter your gentleness in us. In your kind name we ask, AMEN.

- Read Philippians 2:5-11; 2 Corinthians 10:1; Luke 23:39-46.

- Listen to "He Leadeth Me" by iWorship at https://youtu.be/Zwm7MlUtDa0

FOR REFLECTION

In what ways have you observed gentleness or managed to exhibit gentleness during this season?

44

The Lord Is Near

The Lord is near.
Do not be anxious about anything.
PHILIPPIANS 4:5-6, NIV

MAYBE SOMEONE HAS quoted it to you: "Do not be anxious about anything, but in every situation, by prayer and petition, with thanksgiving, present your requests to God." (Philippians 4:6, NIV). This verse offers a hopeful response to anxiety, but sometimes people toss it out flippantly as a quick-fix remedy. When you are confined to a waiting room while your loved one undergoes a five-hour heart surgery, "not being anxious" isn't so simple and straightforward. How can we become "anxious for nothing" as we wait?

As verse six instructs, we can pray and thank God for his love and provision and power. But one of the most compelling reasons for staying calm is actually stated in verse five: "The Lord is near." What does it mean that the Lord is near, or "at hand" as some translations say, and how does this reality bring peace?

To understand how the Lord's nearness brings peace, imagine Baby Jenny screaming for her mom. Aunt Laura picks her up, but Jenny wails more loudly. Jenny's mom returns to the room, takes her from Aunt Laura, and the baby immediately calms. Her mother is near. This scenario reveals three things about the Lord's nearness:

1. It is **the Lord** who is near. Baby Jenny is calmed by her mother's presence because her mom has shown herself to be completely trustworthy. The Lord who is near intricately designed the heart that is being operated on. The Lord who is near sustains the beat of that heart. The Lord who is near loves that heart more than anyone on earth ever could. We are calmed by the Lord who is near because he is our perfect Creator, Sustainer, Redeemer, and Friend.

2. The Lord is **near.** Baby Jenny is comforted by her mom's nearness: she relaxes, recognizing her mom's smell, touch, and voice. The Lord who is near walked the earth as Jesus, God-made-flesh. The Lord who is near fed the multitudes and ate with them; he touched and healed the sick. The Lord who is near bore real scars on his hands when he died for our sins. When Jesus ascended to heaven, he left the Holy Spirit, his presence in us, to comfort us as we wait (John 16:7).

3. The Lord is **near,** that is, "at hand." In other words, he is coming soon. Baby Jenny's mom left the room, but she returned quickly, restoring Jenny's comfort and peace. Jesus is near now through the Holy Spirit, but one day he will return, destroying all disease, defeating evil fully and finally. This anxious season in the waiting room will not go on forever. Dear friends, when you feel the creep of anxiety as you wait, remember the Lord who is so very near.

PRAYER

Lord, thank you for being near to the broken-hearted; for lifting up those who are crushed in spirit (Psalm 34:18). Help us lean into your presence during this anxious wait; calm us with the surpassing peace of Christ. In his ever-near name we pray, AMEN.

FURTHER ENCOURAGEMENT

Read Psalm 118:6; Psalm 145:18; Psalm 34:18.

FOR REFLECTION

What are you facing today that causes you to feel anxious? How does seeing the Lord as near bring peace and hope?

45

Mat-Friends

*....four men arrived carrying a paralyzed man
on a mat. They couldn't bring him
to Jesus because of the crowd, so they dug
a hole through the roof above his head.
Then they lowered the man on the mat,
right down in front of Jesus.*
MARK 2:4, NLT

THE SEASON IN the waiting room can flatten us, strike us down like the paralytic on the mat. In such times, we need faithful friends like those described in this story in Mark. Let's take a look.

Jesus has returned home to Capernaum (the "city of comfort"). The Pharisees, in typical fashion, are hanging around, trying to catch Jesus doing something they think he's not supposed to do. Jesus is preaching to a packed house. And then this strange event occurs.

Four men have decided to take their paralyzed friend to Jesus. The crowd is so thick they can't get through, so they climb the stairs to the roof and dig through the clay tiles, making a hole. Then they lower the man through the hole. He lands at the feet of Jesus. Can you picture this odd scene?

What kind of faith would drive these men to do such a thing? They risked looking ridiculous, angering the homeowner, and/ or being rejected by Jesus and the crowd.

Thankfully, they are neither rejected nor chastised. Jesus heals the man. The reason given for Jesus' healing is intriguing: "*Seeing their faith*, Jesus said to the paralyzed man, 'My child, your sins are forgiven'" (my emphasis, Mark 2:5, NLT). Something about the friends' faith as well as the paralytic's compelled Jesus to heal.

"Mat-friends," driven by their genuine faith in Christ, go to extraordinary lengths to lay the hurting before Jesus. During our season in the waiting room, mat-friends brought us before Jesus in many ways:

- One friend, responding to email prayer requests, wrote out her lovely prayers. Her prayers bundled me up in Scripture and laid me, in my paralyzed emotional state, before Jesus.

- Other friends who lived far away sent a large bouquet of sunflowers, reminding me that God works in ways humans have never imagined (2 Cor. 2:9).

- New friends, who were previously complete strangers, sent cards, treats, books, and entire meals, carrying us with their practical services to the Jesus who tends to us in the flesh (Matthew 25:35-40).

Even when we have mat-friends, we may feel isolated during this season of health crisis. In such times, we can remember the One who burst through a barrier more obstructive than a clay roof to be a friend to us—Jesus himself. Dear friend, will you let Jesus lay you before the Father who cares for you?

Oh, precious Jesus, what a friend we have in you! We thank you also for the mat-friends who have laid us before you throughout our lives and in this season in particular. In your faithfully-loving name we pray, AMEN.

FURTHER ENCOURAGEMENT

- Read Mark 2:1-5; Matthew 25:35-40.
- Listen to "What a Friend We Have in Jesus" by Alan Jackson at https://youtu.be/znWu2HCJ92c

FOR REFLECTION

Make a list of all the people who have shown you acts of kindness during this season. Thank God for how they have revealed Jesus' friendship to you.

46

What Is Healing?

So all of us who have had that veil removed
can see and reflect the glory of the Lord.
And the Lord—who is the Spirit—
makes us more and more like him as we
are changed into his glorious image.
2 CORINTHIANS 3:18

WHILE OUR SON was going through his series of three brain surgeries, my Bible reading was taking me through the first three gospels. Day after day, reading Matthew, Mark, and Luke, I found true stories of Jesus healing the sick, the lame, the blind. One day, finishing my morning devotion in the hospital room where our son was getting a course of IV antibiotics for a bone infection, I got a little fed up.

I prayed, "God, you healed so many people. Why haven't you healed our son?" The answer shot back, Holy-Spirit-sent, "I *have* healed your son." This exchange led me to write in my journal, "What if my idea of healing is being whole physically, but God's main concern is spiritual healing: conforming our son (and us) to the image of Christ?"

In the story of the paralytic, Jesus seems primarily focused on spiritual healing (Mark 2:5-12). The paralytic's friends believe

Jesus can heal his paralysis. Jesus, seeing their faith, says, "Son, your sins are forgiven." Perhaps the mat-friends would like to interject, "But wait, Jesus, what about his physical disability?"

By forgiving the paralytic's sins, Jesus emphasizes that what everyone needs most is spiritual healing. Jesus is not saying that a specific sin caused the man's paralysis. He is demonstrating that the effects of sin and the fall are widespread; they include disease and death. The story teaches several important lessons for those of us in a health crisis:

1. *Do not* assume that a specific sin caused a person's illness; *do* recognize that spiritual healing and physical healing are interrelated.

   About Mark 2:5, Eugene Peterson writes, "The injection of forgiveness into this story shows us something about the rule of God in Christ.... Christ as our King is concerned with our whole lives —with our spiritual paralysis as well as our physical paralysis."[36]

2. Jesus rules over sin and death, spiritual brokenness and physical brokenness.

   The Pharisees are infuriated with Jesus because they think he is equating himself with God—and he is! Jesus proves his authority over the spiritual realm by forgiving sins. Then he demonstrates his power over the physical realm by telling the paralyzed man, "Stand up, pick up your mat, and go home!" (Matthew 9:6, NLT).

3. Jesus' healing, both spiritual and physical, leads people

to glorify God. As the paralyzed man walks out of the crowded hut, we are told, "They were all amazed and praised God, exclaiming, 'We've never seen anything like this before!'" (Mark 2:12, NLT).

As we long and pray for healing, may we see and hear the Jesus who heals the soul even as he heals the body. He rules over us, and he loves us. This is good news indeed.

PRAYER

King Jesus, we praise you, for you rule over all with grace and truth. Forgive our sins, and heal us in heart, soul, mind, and body. In your powerful name, which has all authority in heaven and on earth, AMEN.

FURTHER ENCOURAGEMENT

Read Mark 2:6-12; Psalm 103:3; Isaiah 38:17.

FOR REFLECTION

Write your questions about healing, then lift them to God in prayer.

47

Termites, Tumors, and Other Hidden Dangers

"For he will command his angels concerning
you to guard you in all your ways."
PSALM 91:11, ESV

THREE WEEKS BEFORE our son's fourth brain surgery, we made an unwelcome discovery—termites had eaten through an entire outer wall of our home. We were given only one outward sign of the internal destruction: our son-in-law happened to lean against a wooden windowsill and notice that it seemed hollow.

The hidden termite damage made me think of our son's diagnosis and surgeries. Before he was diagnosed with a low-grade glioma that turned out to be a neuronal dysplasia, he had been performing opera, working eleven and twelve-hour days. He had absolutely no neurological symptoms; his only health problem was chronic sinus congestion, for which he had the CT-scan that revealed the mass in his brain.

After the termite discovery, I began to think about how many hidden dangers lurk in our lives, unseen demons, creating havoc behind the scenes, while we carry on, completely unaware. I realized I could respond to these hidden dangers in one of two ways:

- Option A: I could completely freak out because at any moment a wall that looked perfectly sturdy could collapse on me, or my extremely healthy twenty-two-year-old son could be diagnosed with a brain tumor.

- Option B (much better option!): I could recognize that God has protected us from multitudinous hidden and undisclosed dangers, and I could thank him for his rescue.

The Bible lists numerous ways God rescues us. Here are five:

1. "He rescues you from hidden traps" (Psalm 91:3, MSG). Daily we are confronted with hidden traps that we may never even recognize. Just think about phishing emails and computer hacking attempts. God rescues us from deceit and treachery all of the time, whether we realize it or not.

2. He "shields you from deadly hazards" (Psalm 91:3, MSG). Long ago, a neighbor's child careened down our steep driveway, colliding hard with our brick mailbox. When she stood up, completely unscathed, her mother and I could only conclude that unseen angels had shielded her from harm.

3. He is faithful and "will strengthen you and protect you from the evil one" (2 Thessalonians 3:3, NIV). The devil prowls around like a roaring lion (1 Peter 5:8, NIV); Satan is the father of lies (John 8:44). In our own strength, we would never recognize all of his attempts to ensnare us.

It is the Lord who protects us, moment by moment, day by day.

4. He saves you from condemnation: "And since we have been made right in God's sight by the blood of Christ, he will certainly save us from God's condemnation" (Romans 5:9, ESV). The most serious danger, though not always hidden, is our own deadly sin. Christ has rescued us from God's judgment, giving us everlasting life with God.

PRAYER

Lord, as we read your Word, we discover innumerable reasons for peace and hope during this season. Help us not to fear hidden dangers but to trust in your saving love. In Jesus' rescuing name, AMEN.

FURTHER ENCOURAGEMENT

- Read Psalm 91.

- Listen to "Mighty to Save" by Laura Story at https:// youtu.be/W1jmqVU4RDo

FOR REFLECTION

Make a list of hidden dangers that the Lord might have delivered you from. Thank him for his protection.

NOTES

48

Count Your Losses

You keep track of all my sorrows.
You have collected all my tears in your bottle.
You have recorded each one in your book.
PSALM 56:8, NLT

Missing our daughter's white coat ceremony for PT school.
Cancelling our trip to celebrate our 35ᵗʰ anniversary.
Missing my uncle's funeral.
Caring for my dad in the latter stages of his illness....

ONE DAY I BEGAN listing all the losses I had endured during our season in the waiting room. I didn't even count the profound loss our son endured or all of the losses that affected my husband, our other children, and our extended network of family and friends. During a health crisis, the losses mount like so many soldiers on the beaches of Normandy. Is it appropriate to count them, to take stock of our sorrows?

The Psalmists say, emphatically, *yes.* Of the 150 Psalms, somewhere between 65 and 67 are "psalms of lament," depending on how they are categorized. Asaph, for example, cried: "You don't let me sleep, I am too distressed even to pray! I think of the good old days, long since ended, when my nights were filled with joyful songs…. Has the Lord rejected me forever?" (Psalm 77:4-5a, 7, NLT). And David, the man after God's own heart, moaned, "My eyes are swollen with weeping, waiting for my God to help me…Their insults have broken my heart, and I am in despair. If only one person would show some pity; if only one would turn and comfort me." (Psalm 69:3, 21, NLT).

As each person cries out to God, even as he raises his fist at God as the one responsible for his sorrows, a tectonic shift of the heart occurs. God's unfailing love drives this shift, and the lamenter begins to assert hope in God.

After his outcry, Asaph's focus shifts to God's power: "Oh, God, your ways are holy. Is there any God as mighty as you? You are the God of great wonders! You demonstrate your awesome power among the nations" (Psalm 77:13-14, NLT).

David's heart also changes: "For the Lord hears the cries of the needy; he does not despise his imprisoned people. Praise him O heaven and earth, the seas and all that move in them" (Psalm 69:33-34, NLT).

As we tally our tears, we discover a compassionate God who is counting them right alongside us. The same God who counts our tears sent his Son Jesus to weep human tears for and with us. The same God who counts our tears will one day wipe every one away when Jesus returns to restore all broken things. Remembering God's kindness helps us wait with hope for the day when all losses will be accounted for.

PRAYER

Tear-tracking God, help us to count our losses and to discover your amazing love even as we do. Help us weep tears over our own sin as well as the pain we encounter in a fallen world. In Jesus' compassionate name we pray, AMEN.

FURTHER ENCOURAGEMENT

- Choose one lament Psalm: Psalm 56, 69, or 77, and read it all the way through.

- Listen to "We Will Feast in the House of Zion" by Sandra McCracken at https://youtu.be/ujVBV3lNSbQ.

FOR REFLECTION

Make a list of the losses you have suffered during this season. Ask God to reveal his compassion to you in the midst of such loss.

NOTES

49

Count Your Blessings

For it is all for your sake, so that as grace
extends to more and more people it may
increase thanksgiving, to the glory of God.
2 CORINTHIANS 4:15, ESV

AT TIMES DURING our season in the waiting room, I was far better at counting losses than I was at counting blessings. When things went so far wrong and our son had had three surgeries in four weeks' time, I did not feel very grateful. But I knew the apostle Paul's insistence that God's grace grows a heart of gratitude.

Our sin nature bends our heart away from gratitude in the best of times; during hard seasons, gratitude may take more effort than ever. Author Ann Voskamp, in her pivotal work on gratitude, *One Thousand Gifts*, emphasizes the effort involved when she asks, "How do I see grace, give thanks, find joy in this sin-stinking place?"[37] Indeed, when my eight-three-year-old father was wearing a diaper and moaning in pain, I had to work to see grace, to give thanks.

Gratitude does not deny the painful reality of living in a fallen world; after all, the apostle Paul wrote, "We are pressed on every side by troubles, but we are not crushed. We are perplexed, but not driven to despair. We are hunted down, but never abandoned by God" (2 Corinthians 4:8-9, NLT). And yet, Paul thanked God in the midst of his suffering because more people were discovering God's grace; therefore, more people were thanking God for his gift of forgiveness, and more people were glorifying God (2 Corinthians 4:15).

With Paul's logic in mind, I began to "recount" (*re*-count) all of the "wonderful deeds of the Lord" (Psalm 9:1b, ESV). I brought to mind his blessings, naming them one by one, as the old song suggests:

- Sweet friends paid us a visit today just after the doctor gave us a hard report. Thank you.

- The doctor gave us a good report today. Thank you.

- A smiling stranger on the elevator held the door for me. Thank you.

- A lovely handwritten card arrived in the mail. Thank you.

- Our son knows Jesus Christ as his Lord and Savior. **Thank you!**

As I listed the many kindnesses of God in the midst of this tumultuous season, guess what happened? My heart settled. It seems the apostle Paul, who had been in prison when he wrote the words, "Rejoice in the Lord always; **again**, I say, rejoice," (Phil. 4:4, ESV), knew exactly what he was talking about. He knew that we are made to thank and glorify God; that is the essence of life for a follower of Christ. As we remember the redemption God has worked in our lives, we trust God to work wonders again.

PRAYER

Lord, thank you for your grace, thank you for your Holy Spirit who jogs our memory to "forget not all your benefits." Thank you most of all your Son, our Savior, Jesus Christ, in whose name we pray, AMEN.

FURTHER ENCOURAGEMENT

- Read Psalm 9.

- Listen to "Blessings" by Laura Story at https://youtu.be/JKPeoPiK9XE

FOR REFLECTION

Try keeping a gratitude journal for three days. See Appendix for ideas on creating a gratitude journal.

50

Nothing Can Separate Us

For I am sure that neither death nor life,
nor angels nor rulers, nor things present
nor things to come, nor powers, nor height
nor depth, nor anything else in all
creation, will be able to separate us from
the love of God in Christ Jesus our Lord.
ROMANS 8:38-39, ESV

MY FAMILY LOVES a good roasted chicken. After we have devoured the tasty, moist meat, I strip what is left, throw the bones in a pressure cooker, add some water, and make a rich, nutritious stock. This stock can then season other dishes or deliver healthy nutrients to a frail digestive system. Although we might not expect the bare bones of a chicken to have much to offer, it turns out they do.

In the same way, our lives are sometimes stripped of the "meat," the sweet and tender moments of life that offer comfort. In this bare-bones season, we have the opportunity to discover the essence of what we believe. Our son put words to his bare-bones belief during his third hospital stay.

One night after his third surgery, a group of his friends had gathered in his room. They were passing around the ugly helmet he had been instructed to wear to protect the actual hole in his head. The helmet looked kind of like football headgear from the 1930's and was the color of, as one older gentleman discreetly described it, "dirty diaper brown." We were all laughing at the absurd image of my son walking down the street in such a thing. Suddenly the older gentleman changed the tone, speaking seriously to our son. "If anyone can pull this off, you can. You are amazing."

There was a silence as everyone considered everything our son had been through in the last six weeks and the strong faith with which he had met each challenge. My son spoke,

"Nothing…. nothing…" His voice broke, and a few tears slid down his cheek. "Nothing can take friends and family…." There was another pause, then he finished his thought, "Nothing can take friends and family…and *Jesus*…away from me."

Boom. Mic drop.

In the season of stripping that is a health crisis, this is what we must know. When we can't quite digest the meatier aspects of our theology, we must be "persuaded," as the apostle Paul writes, that "nothing can separate us from the love of God which is in Christ Jesus our Lord" (Romans 8:38, NKJV). *Nothing* can separate us from God's love. *Nothing.*

> Not a terminal diagnosis.
> Not a season of great success at work.
> Not spiritual powers that seek to do harm.
> Not present hardship, nor future prosperity.
> Not "anything else in all creation" (Romans 8:39b, ESV).

Drink deeply, dear friend, of this nourishing stock, and be

strengthened by the preserving love of God in Christ Jesus.

PRAYER

Lord, you know the many things we fear, and you
know the many things we think will bring us life.
Help us to be convinced that your abundant love is
something no one can take from us. Through your
ever-present Spirit we pray, AMEN.

FURTHER ENCOURAGEMENT

Read Romans 8:28-39.

FOR REFLECTION

Make a list of things that feel threatening or frightening to
you today. After you have finished, write above and below the
list, "For I am persuaded that…nothing will be able to separate us from the love of God in Christ Jesus our Lord."

NOTES

51

Return to Normal

*Truly, truly I say to you, unless a grain of
wheat falls into the earth and dies, it remains
alone; but if it dies, it bears much fruit.*
JOHN 12:24, ESV

WHEN OUR SEASON in the waiting room comes to an end,
well-meaning people may say, "Now you can get back to normal." What they may not understand is that we never return
to normal after such suffering; suffering changes us, sometimes for the worse, but usually for the better. As Dr. Gerald
Sittser, who lost his wife, mother, and daughter in a car accident, explains:

> Catastrophic loss by definition precludes recovery.
> It will transform us or destroy us, but it will never
> leave us the same.... One learns the pain of others by
> suffering one's own pain.... The soul is elastic, like a
> balloon. It can grow larger through suffering.[38]

It is such growth through suffering that Jesus describes to
his disciples on the Sunday before his death. He has already
told them that the time has come for him to be glorified (John
12:23). He goes on to explain, "...unless a grain of wheat falls

into the earth and dies, it remains alone; but if it dies, it bears much fruit" (John 12:24, ESV). Just as Jesus had to die and be buried before he was raised from the dead and glorified, so his followers must lose the lives we have loved in this world; in doing so, we gain life for eternity.

For our family, losing the lives we loved in this world meant literally saying good-bye to my father, uncle, and daughter-in-law's grandmother. It also meant surrendering our son's health and life to the Lord. We had learned this lesson of saying, "Not my will, but thine be done" numerous times over the years of raising four children. But this time we were acknowledging that our son's life or death lay in the Lord's hands. As we laid our son on that metaphorical altar, it felt at times as if the darkness would envelop us. And yet, the waiting room season also schooled us in a particular suffering we had not previously known. In this loss, our souls were transformed; our hope was enlarged, and our faith was strengthened.

Indeed, the profound losses of the waiting room may bury us in darkness for a season. By the work of the Holy Spirit, we will one day emerge from the darkness afresh, with bright, green, if somewhat frail at first, leaves unfurling from tender sprouts. One day a bud will appear, and it will mature and become a bright red rose. For this reason, dear friends, don't fret about "returning to normal."

PRAYER

Lord, thank you that we don't "return to normal" after a season in the waiting room. Thank you, Holy Spirit, for taking that buried seed and turning it into a beautiful flower that may point to God's grace and glory. In Jesus' suffering name we pray, AMEN.

- Read John 12:20-26; Romans 6:1-11.

- Listen to "All Things New" by Steven Curtis Chapman at https://youtu.be/FhpQN9JXNXA

FOR REFLECTION

In what ways do you understand the suffering of Christ more fully now? In what ways have you seen Christ's glory in this season?

NOTES

52

A Good Scar Story

....and with his wounds we are healed.
ISAIAH 53:5, ESV

FRIENDS AND I always laugh about the time their eleven-year-old son was forced to make backseat conversation with me during a long drive. My husband and his dad were talking in the front seat, and after thirty minutes of awkward conversation with me, our friends' son suddenly blurted out the question, "So, do you have any good scars?" His dad was mortified, but I found it quite amusing. I understood that to an eleven-year-old boy, a good scar story was the best kind of story. After all, good scar stories point to tragedy, conflict, and ultimately, redemption.

Scars, in their very nature, represent both harm and healing. The flesh has been cut or opened, either on purpose or by accident; a mark remains where the wound has healed. As we look on our loved ones' scars and recall the pain they suffered, we may also remember the physical pain Jesus endured to win the victory over sin and death.

Isaiah 53:5 clearly connects Jesus' suffering with our healing: "But he was pierced for our rebellion, crushed for our sins. He was beaten so we could be whole. He was whipped so we could be healed" (NLT). Consider the physical torment Jesus endured:

- Before Jesus was crucified, he was beaten and then scourged. A scourge was used in ancient times to punish criminals; it inflicted "deep lacerations, torn flesh, and excessive bleeding,"[39] leaving the victim near death.

- A crown of thorns was placed on Jesus' head in mockery. The thorns clawed at his forehead and caused it to bleed.

- Jesus' arms were stretched out and his hands and feet nailed to the cross with thick, six-inch-long nails.

- Hanging from the cross, Jesus would have experienced severe dehydration and ultimately suffocation.

- Even after Jesus died, soldiers stabbed his side with a spear just to make sure he was dead.

Jesus suffered grievous injury on our behalf, and the scars on his resurrection body are a brutal reminder of our sin.

And yet, Jesus' scars also bring rejoicing, because they point us to his victory over sin and death. When Jesus first appeared to the disciples after he was resurrected, John tells us, ".... he showed them the wounds in his hands and in his side. They were filled with joy when they saw the Lord!" (John 20:20, NLT). A few days later, Thomas, who had missed Jesus' first appearance and doubted that it occurred, upon seeing Jesus' scars, cried out in worship, "My Lord and My God!" (John 20:28, ESV). Jesus' scars proved that he really was the risen Lord!

In the same way, while our loved ones' scars may cause us to weep at the sin-marked world, they also lead us to rejoice as we remember the scars of Jesus. Our Lord's scars have won redemption for us and have accomplished healing for all scars—if not now, then certainly in the future.

PRAYER

Dear suffering Lord Jesus, help us to see you in the scars. Help us to remember how deeply you loved us and how hard you fought for us. In your victorious name we pray, AMEN.

FURTHER ENCOURAGEMENT

- Read John 19-20; Isaiah 53.

- Listen to "When I Survey the Wondrous Cross" by Kathryn Scott at https://youtu.be/xLXx2CJ_drs

FOR REFLECTION

Do you have any "good" scar stories? How do they lead you to remember redemption?

53

Grieving in Uncertainty

Will not the Judge of the earth do right?
GENESIS 18:25, ESV

WHEN MY DAD was diagnosed with Stage IV prostate cancer, one source of grief was my fear that he was not a believer. For years I had prayed for his salvation, and whenever I could do so without offending him, I asked about his beliefs. On more than one occasion, he told me that he believed "all roads lead up to the top of the mountain." That sounded to me like a clear denial of Jesus' claim, "I am the way, the truth, and the life. No one comes to the Father except through me" (John 14:6, ESV).

Over the two years that my father lived with cancer, I began to see his heart soften. One day, while waiting to see his oncologist, he was telling me about living in San Diego where his dad was stationed in the navy. He casually mentioned that he had been baptized there as a ten-year-old. Shortly after that, I gave him a Bible, realizing he didn't have one, and he gently teased me about joining me at ladies Bible study. After that, whenever I saw him, he asked me about Thessalonians. And then, as I have mentioned in an earlier meditation ("Do You Believe in Miracles"), we learned that our son did not have cancer, and he sent that famous text, "To God be the glory." Two weeks later, he died.

For years, I had dreaded his death because I had no assurance about whether I would see him in heaven. But now, God gave me a peace. Still no certainty—there was no way I could know for sure. But there was a peace.

Author and theologian Nancy Guthrie points out three major factors to consider as we mourn someone's death whose salvation we are uncertain about:

1. We can never perfectly evaluate another person's heart. We are looking for the fruit that characterizes the life of a believer, but there may be little to none. For example, the only evidence of fruit for the repentant thief on the cross was trusting in Christ just before he died.

2. God is trustworthy. Genesis 18:25 says, "Will not the Judge of all the earth do right?" The answer is "yes." We can trust him to judge fairly.

3. God is rich in mercy. As Guthrie says, "He loves to save. We often have hurdles we want people to jump through to believe that they have been joined to Christ. We are often stingy with mercy."[40]

Dear friends, if you have lost or are facing the loss of a loved one of whose faith you are unsure, I encourage you to grieve with hope in the God who is fair and merciful. Yes, we must wait to see what will be revealed. But we can trust that God is glorious and good, and that He will wipe away all tears in that day.

PRAYER

Holy and just Father, we plead for your mercy regarding our loved ones. Bring them to bow before Jesus as their loving Savior. Give us wisdom and peace as we walk alongside them. In Jesus' redeeming name we pray, AMEN.

FURTHER ENCOURAGEMENT

Read Luke 23:39-43; Ephesians 2:4; Exodus 34:6.

FOR REFLECTION

Do you have concerns about whether your loved one believes? Write a prayer to God asking him to bring you comfort and peace in your grief.

NOTES

54

Do You Believe in Miracles?

*But Jesus rebuked the evil spirit and healed
the boy. Then he gave him back to his father.
Awe gripped the people as they saw this
majestic display of God's power.*
LUKE 9:42-43, NLT

A HEALTH CRISIS often forces us to wrestle with what we
believe about miracles. In Scripture, some miracles center
around supernatural intervention affecting the natural order
of things. These miracles usually point to God's power and
glory. Though such miracles occur today, we may miss them if
we believe only in things we can quantify and explain.

When our son underwent his first brain surgery, we expected
to hear a diagnosis based on the severity of our son's tumor.
But during that surgery, something strange occurred. The
neurosurgeon opened the covering over the brain (the dura)
and saw what appeared to be a malformation of some of the
veins (known as an AV malformation). He and another expert
performed an intracranial ultrasound, and they agreed: they
would not proceed with the surgery at that moment. The
doctor called us out of the waiting room to deliver what he
believed was "very hopeful news"—our son did not have a

brain tumor.

The next day, further testing was done to confirm the diagnosis and determine how to proceed in treating the AV malformation, which can also threaten the brain. But we were now presented with a second shocking reality: that day's tests revealed no evidence of AV malformation.

There were three possible explanations for what had happened:

1. The malformation had been cured when the dura was surgically opened.

2. God had healed the malformation outside of ordinary natural processes.

3. Two surgeons, both brilliant experts in their fields, had been mistaken about their diagnosis.

Ultimately, it was determined that whether or not the AV malformation had ever existed, there was still a tumor that required removal. Another surgery was performed. Even after removing the mass, the neurosurgeon believed it to be a brain tumor, perhaps of a more dangerous sub-type than he had originally feared. However, when a renowned pathologist examined the tissue, he found it to be non-cancerous, a mass of neurons called a "neuronal dysplasia."

If you think this is a bizarre story, you are not alone. Even the medical experts were puzzled. What puzzled me, though, was that none of the medical experts ever mentioned the possibility that something extraordinary had happened. It seemed more likely to me that God had healed in an extraordinary manner than that the veteran doctors had made an incorrect diagnosis.

However the healing occurred, this story encourages us to expand our understanding of how God works healing. As John Stott explains, "*all* healing is divine healing, whether without the use of means or through the use of physical, psychological, or surgical means. The former should probably be termed 'miraculous healing,' while the latter is non-miraculous, but both are equally 'divine healing.'"[41] We may never know whether our son's healing was "miraculous" or "divine"; we do know it pointed to God's glory.

PRAYER

Indeed, God, to you be the glory! Open our eyes to see your extraordinary work in this world, things our minds have not conceived of, our eyes have not seen. In Jesus' extraordinary name we pray, AMEN.

FURTHER ENCOURAGEMENT

Read Luke 1:34-37; Psalm 145:1-7.

FOR REFLECTION

Re-read John Stott's statement about "divine healing" above. In what ways have you seen God work healing in this story? What healing do you still long to see? Share your gratitude and your longings with God.

NOTES

55

Everyday Miracles

Who can list the glorious miracles of the Lord?
Who can ever praise him enough?
PSALM 106:2, NLT

OUR TWENTY-FIRST CENTURY worldview, which tends to believe in things we can quantify and explain, hinders our ability to understand miracles. A biblical worldview, on the other hand, sees all of creation as perpetually dependent on God's creating and sustaining activity. Christ, the visible image of the invisible God, made the things we see and the things we can't see: "*Everything* was created through him and for him" (Col. 1:16, NLT; emphasis mine).

Once we begin to view miracles through a biblical lens, we will observe the Lord's faithful love working in the small and large stories of our lives, and we will praise him for the mercies he has shown. We will join with David, who in Psalm 145, sang, "I will meditate on your majestic, glorious splendor and your wonderful miracles…. Everyone will share the story of your wonderful goodness…" (Psalm 145:5-6, NLT).

We will observe seemingly ordinary events pointing to God's extraordinary goodness:

215

- Finding a parking place in the crowded deck when we're running ten minutes late to our appointment because there was yet another traffic jam on I-65.

- Seating us next to the waiting room angel who a crucial message to share with my father and me (See "Forgiveness").

We will take note of surprising, hard to believe acts of God's provision:

- Selling a house. When my dad's tumors had spread to his hips, compromising his mobility, his house, which was in a disastrous state of disrepair, sold quickly and for a good price, providing funds for an assisted living facility.

- Raising up neurosurgeons. Neurosurgeons have made a conscious choice to train for twelve years after college for the dubious privilege of performing 8-12-hour surgeries, missing many nights of sleep and forgoing hours of quality time with loved ones.

We will be stunned by the wonders of his grace and mercy:

- In making dead men walk. It is actually shocking that my eighty-three-year-old father—or anyone, for that matter—would ever come to know Jesus as Lord and Savior. As Ephesians 2:4-5 explains, our sins had killed off our spirit; we didn't even know it, but we were dead in sin. God, rich in mercy, raised our spirit from the dead through Christ. The impossible was made possible by God's grace.

- In showing us mercy rather than condemnation. We are

awed that God would choose *any of us*, sinners deserving judgment, to lavish with his love and free from the sin that binds us. We wonder that God would bless and multiply his people and fill us with his joy and peace.

The good news of the gospel for us in the waiting room is that we have a creating, sustaining and redeeming God who is working miracles every day, all day. We need only to open our eyes to notice them.

PRAYER

Thank you, Lord of all creation, for working through every story and season of our lives. We praise you for your "glorious splendor" and your "wonderful miracles!" In Jesus' redeeming name we pray, AMEN.

FURTHER ENCOURAGEMENT

- Read Psalm 145.

- Listen to "How Great Is Our God" by Chris Tomlin at https://youtu.be/DpIcqoKOz2M

FOR REFLECTION

List some of the everyday miracles God has worked for you during this season in the waiting room.

56

An Angelic Army

*The angel of the Lord encamps around those
who fear him, and delivers them.*
PSALM 34:7, ESV

UNTIL OUR SEASON in the waiting room, I knew enough about angels in the Bible to realize that they probably didn't look like the petite blond-haired, blue-eyed, cherry-lipped winged figure we propped on the top of my childhood Christmas tree. But I didn't think much about angels interacting with people today on a regular basis. Then, just before our son faced his second surgery, our pastor mentioned in a sermon that God sends angels to guard his people, and I decided to investigate.

As I studied Scripture and commentaries, I learned a lot about angels. Angels are:

- Spiritual beings who were created before humans. They are moral and have free will; thus, they can be tempted, and they can sin (Satan and his fallen angels, Matthew 25:41, 2 Peter 2:4, Revelation 12:9).

- Though angels are spiritual, they do appear in bodily form in the Bible (Genesis 18:2, 16, 22; Acts 27:23).

- When angels appear in bodily form, they often wear white, and they shine with God's glory, with an appearance like lightning (Matthew 28:2, Luke 2:9).

- Much of the time, humans are completely unaware of angels' presence (Hebrews 13:2).

- Faithful angels serve God in numerous ways; they can act as messengers (Luke 1:28), ministers of the gospel (Luke 15:10), and mighty protectors (Daniel 6:22). As John Piper explains about angels who serve God, "All angels serve for the good of all Christians all the time. They are agents of Romans 8:28."[42]

As I discovered more about the angels of the Bible, God prepared me to rely on this powerful army when I needed it the most. One night before our son's third surgery, I felt the darkness of evil assailing my mind with fearful imaginings of what might happen. I don't know if I was asleep or awake when I called out to the Lord for protection. I do recall a dream in which a large army of angels descended and surrounded my enemies. There was a battle, and then the evil was gone. I felt certain of one thing when I awoke the next morning: a spiritual battle for my mind had occurred, and God had commanded his angels to guard me and restore my peace (Psalm 91:11).

In this season of health crisis, we need to recognize angels as something far more fierce than a blond-haired, blue-eyed doll. We are in a spiritual battle as well as a physical one, and our powerful God has sent his angelic armies to our aid. Take comfort, dear friends, in the Lord's messengers of glory and mighty protectors of body and spirit.

PRAYER

Lord, thank you for loving us so much that you command angelic armies to minister to and protect us. Help us hear your angels singing your glory; help us join with them in praising your name. AMEN

FURTHER ENCOURAGEMENT

Read Matthew 28:2; Hebrews 13:2; Daniel 10.

FOR REFLECTION

What do you know about angels? Have you learned more about angels from Scripture or cultural sources? Have you considered that angels may be protecting and helping you in your current story?

NOTES

57

Tough Decisions

*For the LORD gives wisdom; from His mouth
come knowledge and understanding.*
PROVERBS 2:6, ESV

SHOULD I TAKE my confused father's car keys? Is my mother still able to live on her own, or does she need full-time caregiving? Does she have any express wishes for end-of-life arrangements? And this—one of the hardest questions of all—should we allow the medical staff to turn on (or off) life support? The wide array and heavy weight of the crucial decisions facing us in the waiting room can be bewildering. We need not be dismayed; God has provided many excellent resources for gaining the wisdom we so desperately need:

1. Seek help from the Holy Spirit in fervent prayer, inviting others to pray with and for you (James 1:5). The Lord may answer your prayers by directing you to Scripture, or he may lead you to people who can provide knowledgeable counsel.

2. Seek wisdom in Scripture as you discuss end-of-life decisions. Dr. Bill Davis, in his fine work, *Departing in Peace: Biblical Decision-Making and the End of Life*, offers three

foundational biblical principles to consider. He explains that God's Word...

- "obligates us to protect and nurture human life."[43]

- "teaches that long physical life is a great good, but it is not the highest biblical good." [44]

- "assures us that death is a great evil, but it is not the ultimate evil...."[45]

3. Seek help from wise Christians who have cared for loved ones in health crises. They will often know of excellent resources; they also will understand your commitment to honor God in your decisions. One friend explained the need to have my dad's advanced directive on hand; another shared how hospice had helped her dad at the end of his life.

4. Seek help from medical experts and caregiving specialists. Although the attending physician may not always be accessible, nurses, palliative care specialists, chaplains and social workers can all provide valuable information. When we were trying to choose the best type of device for dispensing our son's IV antibiotics, both a nurse and a social worker helped us by explaining the pros and cons of each device.

5. Rest in God's forgiveness and contra-conditional love. You will make mistakes. My dad's condition deteriorated so rapidly that we weren't able to get hospice help for his final days. I felt deeply responsible for the suffering he experienced at the end. After my dad died, his oncologist

gently reminded me, "Your father would not have wanted you to have regrets. He knew you were caring for your son, and that was your dad's priority and yours."

Indeed, the burden of regret is too heavy for any human. In these heartrending decisions, dear friends, we can and must run to and rest in Jesus, who has the ultimate power over life and death.

PRAYER

Lord, help. By your Spirit, teach us your Word and give us your wisdom to make life-altering decisions for and with those we love. In Jesus' all-wise name we pray, AMEN.

FURTHER ENCOURAGEMENT

- Read Psalm 91:1, 16; Isaiah 25:6-8; Ecclesiastes 3:1-8.

- Listen to "The Perfect Wisdom of our God" by Keith and Kristyn Getty at https://youtu.be/hSnzYnOe6kI

FOR REFLECTION

Consider the three biblical principles mentioned by Dr. Bill Davis (see above). How might any or all of these apply to a decision you currently need to make?

58

The First Enemy: Satan

Stay alert! Watch out for your great enemy, the
devil. He prowls around like a roaring lion,
looking for someone to devour.
1 PETER 5:8, NLT

IT WAS FIVE DAYS after my dad had died. During the past month, I had been slammed by wave after wave of health care needs for our son and my dad:

- Administer our son's IV dose at 5 a.m., 1 p.m., and 9 p.m..

- Run over to the assisted living facility to check on my dad who was now incoherent from his fentanyl patch.

- Talk to home health care about our son's meds.

- Return a call to a different home health care about my dad.

I was floundering.

In retrospect it is little wonder that my husband and I turned on each other like dogs snapping over food the night we learned that our son was immunosuppressed. We were both fried with exhaustion, fear, and deep sorrow. And the devil was prowling around, waiting to pounce, eager to tear us limb by limb and feed on the spoils.

One of the worst mistakes we can make as believers is to ignore or underestimate the very real spiritual power of the "father of lies," (John 8:44, NIV), Satan. In the words of theologian Cornelius Plantinga, Satan "… is a figure who deceives, accosts, seduces, accuses, and destroys—a figure of such power and wiliness that New Testament writers grudgingly title him 'the prince of demons' (Matt. 12:24, RSV), or even 'the god of this world' (2 Cor. 4:4; Jn. 12:31).[46] The devil may attack us in many ways during a health crisis:

- He may attempt to undermine our trust in God as he did with Adam and Eve.

- He may seek to distract us from looking for the hope of Christ in our desperate circumstances.

- He may accuse and shame us, knowing that in this season, we may feel guilt over failures to love our precious ones well.

The good news of the gospel is that Christ has triumphed over Satan (Col. 2:15), and one day Christ will cast him into the pit of hell where he belongs (Revelation 20:10). Meanwhile, God has equipped us by the power of the Holy Spirit to battle against Satan's evil schemes. Ephesians 6:10-18 describes our arsenal:

- Truth, righteousness in Christ, and gospel peace: defends against the lies Satan tells.

- Assurance of salvation: strengthens us against Satan's

condemning accusations.

- Strong faith: reminds us that the God who has begun a good work in us will complete it (Phil. 1:10).

- God's word and strengthening prayer: ultimately slays the mighty dragon Satan and sends him to his certain doom.

Yes, dear friends, our enemy the devil prowls around us, but rest assured, our mighty warrior Jesus has already secured the win.

PRAYER

Prince of Peace, we call on you to defeat the "prince of demons" this very day in this very place. Help us resist his ploys, his seduction to sin, so that we might rest in your overpowering love even now. In your triumphant name we pray, AMEN.

FURTHER ENCOURAGEMENT

- Read Ephesians 6:10-18; Colossians 2:15; Revelation 20:10.

- Listen to "A Mighty Fortress Is Our God" by Chris Rice at https://www.youtube.com/watch?v=bONV_YZCKdg

FOR REFLECTION

Can you identify ways the devil has tried to lure you into sin during this season? What tools have helped you to defend against his schemes?

59

The Final Enemy: Death

The last enemy to be destroyed is death.
1 CORINTHIANS 15:26, ESV

MY DAD, A SCHOLAR of seventeenth-century British litera-
ture, often taught and always appreciated the works of John
Donne. As my dad was dying, lines from Donne's Holy
Sonnet X, "Death Be Not Proud," played in my mind. In the
sonnet, Donne takes death down a notch, reminding death
that though some may think it "mighty and dreadful," it does
not have the last word:

> One short sleep past, we wake eternally,
> And death shall be no more;
> Death, thou shalt die.[47]

John Donne knew what the Bible affirms: death, while a
mighty and dreadful enemy, has lost its power over us. As
Christians, we take comfort from a biblical view of death,
which holds together two seemingly opposed realities:

1. Death is our enemy. When God created the world, he
   intended that humans would live forever, glorifying and
   enjoying him. When sin entered the world, death came

alongside it, separating our souls from God. The devil has used the power of death to hold God's people in bondage to fear ever since (Hebrews 2:15).

2. Death has lost its sting for followers of Christ. When Christ succumbed to death on the cross, he defeated sin, and he defeated death with it. This is why we can join with John Donne and the apostle Paul in mocking the fallen tyrant, death:

> "O death, where is your victory?
> O death, where is your sting?"
> (1 Corinthians 15:55, ESV)

Because Christ was raised from the dead, we too, will be raised with him in glory after death. For the Christian, both life and death are good news. As the apostle Paul said, "For me to live is Christ, and to die is gain" (Phil. 1:21) and, "My desire is to depart and be with Christ, for that is far better" (Phil. 1:23, ESV). Death is no longer bad news for Christians.

What does that mean for us as our loved ones potentially face imminent death? How do we respond? Again, we hold the two seemingly opposing realities together:

1. We fight death with the appropriate means: prayer, medical and technological resources, and wise counsel.

2. We face death on behalf of our loved ones with faith, hope and love.

Sadly, many Christians with terminal diagnoses suffer because their family and friends refuse to engage the reality of their approaching death. Instead, as those who believe that death is the doorway into new life forever with the Father, Son, and Holy Spirit, we can release our tight grip on life here and look forward to life in the hereafter.

One day, the day we most eagerly await, Christ will return. In that day, "He will swallow up death forever; and the Lord God will wipe away tears from all faces…." (Isaiah 25:8, ESV). Until that day comes, we are well-equipped to face death with the hope of resurrection. May this good news bring you great comfort!

PRAYER

Lord, you have said that you would walk alongside us as we enter the valley of the shadow of death. We ask for your strength, hope, and love in these hard days. In Jesus' resurrecting name we pray, AMEN.

FURTHER ENCOURAGEMENT

- Read 1 Corinthians 15:12-58.

- Listen to "Death Be Not Proud" by Audrey Assad at https://youtu.be/9ID7dmCiAgw

FOR REFLECTION

Write a prayer expressing your thoughts and feelings about death. Ask the Lord to meet you wherever you are and to bring you peace.

NOTES

60

The Wait Is Over!

He will wipe away every tear from their eyes,
and death shall be no more, neither shall there
be mourning, nor crying, nor pain anymore,
for the former things have passed away.
REVELATION 21:4, ESV

IT WAS MAY 14, the day of the final re-check after our son's fourth, and Lord-willing, final brain surgery. His neurosurgeon entered the room and smiled broadly when he saw his patient looking so healthy and tanned. After a brief neuro exam, the doctor asked our son about his plans for the near future and then sent him on his way, saying, "I'll see you in December."

December. That was seven months away! After nine months of four surgeries, four recoveries, multiple challenges, numerous CT-scans, MRI's, lab work, and doctor's visits, could we really be done? Was our time in the waiting room over? Could we really celebrate some good news? I was giddy at the thought, but our son was still not sure. Too many things had gone wrong in the past.

Our son's reticence to celebrate is understandable. We live in the season of biblical history sometimes called the "already-not yet." Christ has come, died, and risen from the dead. Those who have trusted him as Savior are united to him, living in the freedom for which he set us free. And yet, we still bear the pain of living in a fallen world. Loved ones die, even when we are declared healthy and fit after a long battle. Even as I celebrated our son's good prognosis, I mourned my father's, my uncle's, and my daughter-in-law's grandmother's deaths. That is the nature of life in this season of our story.

One day, though, the already-not yet will give way to "It is finished!" (Rev. 21:6a, NLT). One day our wait will truly be over. The Bible tells us that Christ will return, and he will make everything new (Revelation 21:5). In that day, God will dwell with his people (Revelation 21:4): we will never feel separated from him as our son did during the almost-four-hour MRI (See "When You Are Lonely"). Our vision, now dimmed by the fall, will in that day, be fully corrected, and we will see Christ "as he really is" (1 John 3:2, NLT). In that day, we will struggle with sin no more, for we will be like him. And, in that day, as Sally Lloyd-Jones puts it in *The Jesus Storybook Bible*, "No more being sick or dying. Because all those things are gone…Everything sad has come untrue."[48]

Today, as we await that wonderful day, we listen for Jesus' voice, calling to us, "Yes, I am coming soon!" And we join the chorus of God's people, "Amen! Come, Lord Jesus!" (Rev. 22:20, NLT).

PRAYER

Lord Jesus, thank you for this season in the waiting room! It has only increased our eagerness to see you again! Come quickly, we pray, and in the meantime, help us to wait with our eyes fixed on the day when you will fully and finally heal all broken things. In your restoring name we pray, AMEN.

FURTHER ENCOURAGEMENT

- Read Revelation 21 and 22.

- Listen to "Great Rejoicing" by Rain for Roots at https:// rainforroots.bandcamp.com/track/great-rejoicing

FOR REFLECTION

Read through Revelation 21 and 22 several times. List some things that you look forward to about the day Jesus returns. Then, write or say a prayer to God about your longing for this final day.

Acknowledgments

In memory of...
Robert Charles Reynolds, Sr.

This book was borne out of many losses and much greater gains. I am indebted to...

My Lord and Savior Jesus Christ.

My husband, Kirby Loftin Turnage III, my faithful companion through many seasons of loss and joy.

Our children and their spouses for your strong faith and deep compassion through this season—we are grateful for how God has worked in your lives to mature and complete you.

> Robert Reynolds Turnage
> Mary Elizabeth and Caleb Blake
> Jackie and Matt Roelofs
> Kirby and Amy Anne Turnage

Our parents for your loving support: Jackie Reynolds, Kirby and Joy Turnage.

Pastoral friends who shepherded us along the rocky path: Scotty and Darlene Smith, Hope Parker, Cheryl Simcox, Christie Tilley, Mary Baker, and Joel and Kate Treick.

A veritable army of prayer warriors and kind friends, including Anne Henegar, Suzy Marshall, Cindy Jank, Susan Calderazzo, Patti McMilion, Dan and Becky Allender, the body of our local church: Pinewoods Presbyterian, the body of our son's college home church: Homewood Cumberland Presbyterian, Samford University and Dean Joseph Hopkins. And to the many prayer warriors unknown to me but known to God, thank you!

The highly accomplished and genuinely caring medical staff at UAB Hospital and The Woodlands Medical Center, especially the Neuro-ICU nurses and staff, as well as Dr. James Markert, Jr., Emily Stewart, P.A., Dr. Esther Dupépé, Dr. Burt Nabors, Dr. Frank Greskovich, III, and Dr. Alejandro Inclan.

The team that helped shape the beauty of this book for my readers:

Editor Kate Treick: for helping me to fashion these words into a story that tells God's glory!

Cover and Interior Designer Erik M. Peterson: for engaging with the story and sharing it through your splendid artistic creation.

Charity Walton of Good Shepherd Publications: for so carefully composing each page for final publication.

Appendix

BOOKS, ARTICLES, AND VIDEOS

The Heidelberg Catechism at TheHeidelbergCatechism.com,
  http://www.heidelberg-catechism.com/en/lords-days/1.
  html

William Davis at http://byfaithonline.com/
  departing-in-peace-making-wise-end-of-life-decisions/

William Davis, Departing in Peace: Biblical Decision-
  Making and the End-of-Life (Phillipsburg, NJ: P & R
  Publishing, 2017).

Sally Balch Hurme, ABA/AARP Checklist for My Family: A
  Guide to My History, Financial Plans and Final Wishes 1st
  Edition (Chicago: American Bar Association, 2015).

Dr. Gerald Sittser, "Adversity as Spiritual Formation" at
  https://cct.biola.edu/adversity-spiritual-formation/

RELAXATION ACTIVITIES

BREATHING

Breathing techniques have been shown to reduce anxiety and
  stress. Try one of these techniques from the University of

Michigan Health Library.

WALKING

Exercise has been shown to alleviate the stress caregivers
often experience. A ten-minute walk outside the hospital
or home benefits the caregiver. For more information, see
Exercise and Caregiving.

MUSIC

For a complete song list, see below. For playlists, please visit
The Waiting Room page at www.elizabethturnage.com/
thewaitingroom.

COLORING AND ART

WEBSITES WITH FREE COLORING PAGES

Karla Dornacher: https://www.karladornacher.com/freebies/

God's Fingerprints: https://godsfingerprints.co/blogs/
blog/3-creative-ways-to-use-your-bible-coloring-pages

BIBLE/ART JOURNALING BOOKS AND WEBSITES

Sue Kemnitz: *Honoring the Spirit* and https://suekemnitz.
com

Anita C. Haines: *Trusting in God*

Karla Dornacher: *Everlasting Hope*

COLORING APPS

Note, these are free trials for seven days, then there is a
charge. Be sure to cancel if you don't want to pay the subscription fee! Pigment and Colorfy are highly rated on both
iTunes and Google.

PIGMENT

Free at iTunes store and Google Play for seven days, then
auto-renewing subscription.

COLORFY

Free at iTunes store and Google play for seven days, then
auto-renewing subscription.

GRATITUDE JOURNALS

Keeping a gratitude journal can be as simple as making a list
of things you are thankful for. Check out the following
resources as well as *The Waiting Room* website or Pinterest
board for more prompts and ideas:

FREE PRINTABLE GRATITUDE JOURNAL

https://www.elizabethturnage.com/thewaitingroom

30 GRATITUDE JOURNAL PROMPTS

http://textmyjournal.com/gratitude-journal-prompts/

GRATITUDE JOURNALS FOR PURCHASE

Brenda Nathan: *Gratitude Journal: A Journal Filled with Favorite Bible Verses*

Ben Greenfield: *Christian Gratitude Journal*: masculine gratitude journal and planner.

CAREGIVER RESOURCES

1. National Caregivers Library

2. AARP Caregiving

3. Caregiver Action Network

Notes

1   G.G. Cohen, R. L. Harris, G. L. Archer Jr., & B. K. Waltke (Eds.), *Theological Wordbook of the Old Testament* (Chicago: Moody Press, 1999), (electronic ed., 875).

2   *The Heidelberg Catechism, Question 1*, at TheHeidelbergCatechism.com, http://www.heidelberg-catechism.com/en/lords-days/1.html. Accessed September 5, 2018.

3   *Heidelberg Catechism, Answer #1*.

4   Ibid.

5   Dietrich Bonhoeffer, ed. Eberhard Bethge, *Letters and Papers from Prison* (New York, N.Y.: MacMillan Publishing Company, 1971), 347.

6   "Believe." Merriam-Webster.com, *Merriam-Webster*, www.merriam-webster.com/dictionary/believe. Accessed January 8, 2018.

7   Dan Allender and Tremper Longman III. *Cry of the Soul* (Colorado Springs: NavPress, 1994), 155.

8   Eugene Peterson, *Answering God* (New York, NY: HarperCollins, 1991), 91-92.

9   Susan Calderazzo, personal email to author, October 6, 2017.

10 Nancy Guthrie, *The One Year Book of Hope* (Carol Stream, IL: Tyndale, 2005), 171.

11 Eugene Peterson, *Conversations: The Message with Its Translator* (Colorado Springs: NavPress, 2007), 733.

12 Amy Carmichael, *Whispers of His Power* (CLC Publications: Ft. Washington, PA, 1982), 266.

13 Tony Reinke," What We Learn from Nude Reality TV," DesiringGod.com, August 9, 2014, https://www.desiringgod.org/articles/what-we-learn-from-nude-reality-tv. Accessed March 22, 2018.

14 Carmen Imes, "Unanswered Prayer: A Lesson from the Psalms," The Well.inter-varsity.org, November 4, 2016, https://thewell.intervarsity.org/spiritual-formation/unanswered-prayer-lesson-psalms. Accessed May 31, 2018.

15 J.I. Packer, in interview with Ivan Mesa, J. I. Packer, 89, "On Losing Sight But Seeing Christ," Gospel Coalition, January 14, 2016, https://www.

thegospelcoalition.org/article/j-i-packer-89-on-losing-sight-but-seeing-christ/. Accessed May 2, 2018.

16 "Prove." Merriam-Webster.com, *Merriam-Webster*, www.merriam-webster.com/dictionary/prove. Accessed March 22, 2018.

17 Robert K. Brown and Mark R. Norton (Eds.), *The One Year Book of Hymns: 365 Devotional Readings Based on Great Hymns of the Faith* (Wheaton, Il.:Tyndale House, 1995), September 11.

18 Scotty Smith, "A Prayer for the Discouraged," The Gospel Coalition, July 17, 2014, https://www.thegospelcoalition.org/blogs/scotty-smith/a-prayer-for-the-discouraged-4/. Accessed June 28, 2018.

19 Martin Luther, James Galvin (Gen. Ed.) "Our Counselor," in *Faith Alone: A Daily Devotional* (Grand Rapids: Zondervan, 2005), August 16.

20 Scotty Smith, *Notes on John*, in *The Gospel Transformation Bible* (Wheaton, Il.: Crossway, 2013), 1437.

21 John Stott, *The Message of Romans* (Downer's Grove, Il.: InterVarsity Press, 1994), 242.

22 Julian of Norwich, *Revelations of Divine Love*, translated by Grace Warrick (1901), accessed at http://www.ccel.org/ccel/julian/revelations.xiv.i.html on July 20, 2018.

23 Horatio Spafford, "It Is Well with My Soul," in *The One Year Book of Hymns*, ed. Robert K. Brown and Mark R. Norton (Wheaton: Tyndale, 1995), Feb. 4.

24 Mary Bowley Peters, "Through the Love of God Our Savior," at https://hymnary.org/text/through_the_love_of_god_our_savior, accessed July 20, 2018.

25 Paul Miller, *Love Walked among Us: Learning to Love like Jesus* (Colorado Springs: NavPress, 2001), 31.

26 Cornelius Plantinga, *Not the Way It's Supposed to Be: A Breviary of Sin* (Grand Rapids, MI: Wm. B. Eerdmans, 1995), 10.

27 Jerry Sittser, e-mail message to author, April 5, 2018.

28 Paul Tripp, *New Morning Mercies* (Wheaton, Il.: Crossway, 2014), April 9.

29 Amie Patrick, "Self-Care and Self-Denial," The Gospel Coalition, August 10, 2015, https://www.thegospelcoalition.org/article/self-care-and-self-denial/. Accessed June 15, 2018.

30 Frederick Buechner, "Message in the Stars," in *The Magnificent Defeat* (New York: Harpercollins, 1966), 50.

31 Dan Doriani, R. D. Phillips, P. G. Ryken, & D. M. Doriani (Eds.), *Matthew, Vol. 2* (Phillipsburg, NJ: P&R Publishing, 2008), Vol. 2, 17.

32 "Prodigal." Merriam-Webster.com. *Merriam-Webster*, 23 Mar. 2018.

33 Scotty Smith, "Notes on John" in *Gospel Transformation Bible* (Wheaton, Il.: Crossway, 2013), 1429.

34 Amy Carmichael, 258.

35 Carmichael, 258.

36 Peterson, *Conversations*, 1545.

37 Ann Voskamp, *One Thousand Gifts* (Grand Rapids, MI, 2010), 125.

38 Jerry Sittser, *A Grace Disguised* (Grand Rapids: Zondervan, 2004), 73.

39 "The Roman Scourge" at Bible History Online, https://www.bible-history.com/past/flagrum.html. Accessed December 20, 2018.

40 Nancy Guthrie, "Comfort When an Unbeliever Dies," The Gospel Coalition, May 30, 2017, https://www.thegospelcoalition.org/article/comfort-when-unbeliever-dies/. Accessed June 20, 2018.

41 John Stott, *Baptism and Fullness* (Downer's Grove: IVP, 1976), p. 386.

42 John Piper, "The Surprising Role of Guardian Angels," DesiringGod.com, April 4, 2017, https://www.desiringgod.org/articles/the-surprising-role-of-guardian-angels. Accessed May 14, 2018.

43 Bill Davis, *Departing in Peace: Biblical Decision-Making and the End-of-Life* (Phillipsburg, NJ: P & R Publishing, 2017), 38.

44 Davis, 39.

45 Davis, 40.

46 Plantinga, 74.

47 John Donne, "Death Be Not Proud," Poetry Foundation, https://www.poetryfoundation.org/poems/44107/holy-sonnets-death-be-not-proud. Accessed July 2, 2017.

48 Sally Lloyd-Jones, *The Jesus Storybook Bible* (Grand Rapids: Zonderkidz, 2007), 347.

Scripture Index

Genesis

1-3—Introduction. xvii

18:2, 16, 22—An Angelic Army. 219

18:25—Grieving in Uncertainty. 207

50:20—Your Troubled Heart. 35

Exodus

8:2-3—Live by Every Word. 31

15:1-18—Sharing the Story 39

34:6—Grieving in Uncertainty. 207

Numbers

20:12—Looking for a Better Place. 47

Deuteronomy

8:3—Live by Every Word 31

30:11-14—Live by Every Word 31

Joshua

4:1-7—Searching for Signs of
Redemption. 127

6:1-6, 20—Live by Every Word. 31

Job

1-2—Our Ultimate Question. 51

2:9—Our Ultimate Question 51

3:25—Our Ultimate Question 51

12:10—Your Only Comfort 1

13:3, 15—How to Pray; Our Ultimate
Question. 19, 51

19:25—God's Answer 55

38:1-3—God's Answer 55

38-42—God's Answer. 55

40:3-4—God's Answer. 55

42:5—God's Answer 55

Psalms

19:1-6—Searching for Signs of
Redemption. 127

27:13—Never Give Up. 103

30:5—Jesus Wept 159

34:7—An Angelic Army 219

34:18—The Lord Is Near 171

56:8—Count Your Losses 187

69—Count Your Losses 187

77—Count Your Losses 187

78—Sharing the Story. 39

88—Normal Grief. 71

91:1, 16—An Angelic Army 219

91—Termites, Tumors, and Other Hidden
Dangers .183

103:3—What Is Healing? 179

103:13-14—God Knows You. 27

106:2—Everyday Miracles 215

118:6—The Lord Is Near 171

145—Sharing the Story; Everyday
Miracles 39, 215

145:1-7—Do You Believe in Miracles? . .211

145:18—The Lord Is Near 171

Proverbs

2:6—Tough Decisions 223

3:5-6—Knowledge That Will Change
Your World 23

Ecclesiastes

3:1-8—Tough Decisions. 223

Isaiah

3:10—All Will Be Well 95

25:6-8—Tough Decisions; The Final Enemy:
Death. 223, 231

26:3, 12—The Peace of God 111

38:17—What Is Healing?. 179

40:31 — Prayer Requests: Inviting
Community to Pray 43
41:10 — Don't Panic—He's Got You 15
43:1-3 — God Knows You 27
43:7 — Introduction xx
43:9-20 — Knowledge That Will Change Your
World. 23
44:17, 20, 24 — Knowledge That Will Change
Your World 23
53:5 — A Good Scar Story. 203
53:4-5 — Introduction xvii
61:1-3 — Searching for Signs of Redemption.
127
63:7-9 — Worth Waiting For 163
65:17-25 — Worth Waiting For. 163

Jeremiah

29:1-11 — Change of Plans. 75
29:12 — How to Pray. 19

Lamentations

2:19-20 — Steadfast 139
3:1-33 — Steadfast 139

Daniel

6:22 — An Angelic Army 219
10 — An Angelic Army 219

Nahum

1:7-8 — God Knows You 27

Zephaniah

3:17 — Live by Every Word 31

Matthew

5:4 — Jesus Wept 159
9:6 — What Is Healing? 179
10:29-31 — God Rules Everything. 11
11:28-30 — Self-Care: Your Body Is a
Temple. 123
12:24 — The First Enemy: Satan 227

14:22-33 — When You Mistake Jesus
for a Ghost; Jesus Has His Eyes
on You 135, 143
25:31-46 — The Kindness of Strangers; Mat-
Friends 147, 175
25:35-40 — Mat-Friends. 175
25:41 — An Angelic Army 219
26:36-46 — When God Said "No" 131
27:45-50 — When You Are Lonely. 83
28:2 — An Angelic Army 219

Mark

2:1-5 — Mat-Friends 175
2:5-12 — What Is Healing? 179

Luke

1:28 — An Angelic Army 219
1:34-37 — Do You Believe in Miracles? . .211
2:9 — An Angelic Army. 219
5:16 — Self-Care: Your Body Is a
Temple. 123
8:42-48 — Comfort as You Have Been
Comforted 59
9:42-43 — Do You Believe in Miracles? . .211
13:34 — God Knows You. 27
15:10 — An Angelic Army 219
15:11-31 — The Embrace of the Father . .151
22:39-46 — When God Said "No" 131
23:32-34 — When You Are Lonely 83
23:39-43 — Grieving in Uncertainty 207
23:39-46 — The Gentleness of Jesus. . . .167

John

2:1 — Self-Care: Your Body Is a Temple . .123
8:44 — Termites, Tumors, and Other
Hidden Dangers; The First Enemy:
Satan. 183, 227
11:1-37 — The Wrong Question 155
11:17-53 — Jesus Wept 159

12:20-26—Return to Normal 199

12:31—The First Enemy: Satan 227

13:36-14:7—Your Troubled Heart 35

14:6—Grieving in Uncertainty. 207

14:16—Your Helper Is Here 87

14-17—Your Troubled Heart; My Peace

    I Give. 35, 107

14:27—My Peace I Give 107

16:5-15—Your Helper Is Here 87

16:7—The Lord Is Near 171

19:17-27—Loss of Dignity 67

19:30—When You Are Lonely 83

19-20—A Good Scar Story. 203

20:19—My Peace I Give 107

Acts

17:27-28—Your Only Comfort. 1

27:23—An Angelic Army 219

Romans

1:19—Searching for Signs of

    Redemption. 127

2:4—Patience and Patients. 99

5:2-4—All Will Be Well. 95

5:3-5—Becoming Mature and Complete . . 7

5:9—Termites, Tumors, and Other Hidden

    Dangers 183

5:10—My Peace I Give 107

5:12—Introduction xvii

6:1-11—Return to Normal 199

8:18-19—Introduction xvii

8:18-25—Unfulfilled. 91

8:25—Patience and Patients. 99

8:26, 34—Prayer Requests: Inviting

    Community to Pray 43

8:26-27—Your Helper Is Here! 87

8:28—An Angelic Army; My Peace I

    Give. 219, 107

8:28-39—Nothing Can Separate Us. . . .195

8:32—The Embrace of the Father 151

10:8-10—Live by Every Word 31

14:7-8—Your Only Comfort 1

15:1-3—Comfort as You Have Been

    Comforted. 59

1 Corinthians

6:19-20—Your Only Comfort 1

6:20—Self-Care: Your Body Is a

    Temple. 123

13:7—The Community of Faith 115

15:19-21—Unfulfilled 91

15:12-58—The Final Enemy: Death 231

2 Corinthians

1:3-7—Comfort as You Have Been Comforted

    59

3:17-18—Your Helper Is Here! 87

4:4—The First Enemy: Satan 227

4:8-15—Count Your Blessings 191

5:21—My Peace I Give 107

10:1—The Gentleness of Jesus 167

12:7-10—When You Are Weak 119

Galatians

3:29—When God Said "No". 131

5:1—Introduction. xvii

5:22—Patience and Patients. 99

6:2—Self-Care: Your Body Is a Temple . .123

Ephesians

1:7—You Are Forgiven. 3

2:4—Grieving in Uncertainty. 207

2:4-5—Everyday Miracles 215

2:8—'Tis So Sweet to Trust in Jesus. . . . 79

2:14-17—My Peace I Give 107

4:1-3—Patience and Patients 99

6:10-18—The First Enemy: Satan 227

Philippians

1:6—Change of Plans 75
1:10—The First Enemy: Satan 227
2:5-11—When You Are Weak; The Gentleness
    of Jesus 119, 167
3:8-11—All Will Be Well 95
4:4—Count Your Blessings 191
4:5—The Gentleness of Jesus 167
4:5-6—The Lord Is Near 171
4:5-7—Don't Panic—He's Got You 15
4:4-7—The Peace of God 111

Colossians

1:16—Everyday Miracles 215
2:15—The First Enemy: Satan 227
3:15—The Peace of God . . . . —111

1 Thessalonians

5:14—The Community of Faith 115

2 Thessalonians

1:3-12—Becoming Mature and Complete . 7
3:3—Termites, Tumors, and Other Hidden
    Dangers .183

1 Timothy

1:16—Patience and Patients 99
2:1—Prayer Requests: Inviting Community
    to Pray 43

2 Timothy

1:8-14—I Know Whom I Have Believed . . 63

Hebrews

2:9-10—Loss of Dignity 67
2:15—The Final Enemy: Death 231
4:15—Jesus Wept 159
4:28-29—Don't Panic—He's Got You 15
7:25—Prayer Requests: Inviting Community
    to Pray 43
10:24-25—The Community of Faith 115

11:1-12:2—Looking for a Better Place . . 47
12—Loss of Dignity 67
12:2—When God Said "No" 131
13:2—The Kindness of Strangers;
    An Angelic Army 147, 219

James

1:2-4—Becoming Mature and Complete . . 7
1:5—Tough Decisions 223
5:13—How to Pray 19
5:13-16—Prayer Requests: Inviting
    Community to Pray 43

1 Peter

1:18—You Are Forgiven 3
4:13—Live by Every Word 31
4:12-19—'Tis So Sweet to Trust in
    Jesus 79
5:7—The Peace of God 111
5:8—The First Enemy: Satan; Termites,
    Tumors, and Other Hidden
    Dangers 227, 183

2 Peter

2:4—An Angelic Army 219

1 John

1:7—You Are Forgiven 3
2:2—You Are Forgiven 3
3:2—Introduction xvii
3:2—Change of Plans; The Wait Is
    Over! 75, 235

Revelation

12:9—An Angelic Army 219
20:10—The First Enemy: Satan 227
21-22—The Wait Is Over! 235
21:3-4—Introduction xvii
21:4-6—The Wait Is Over! 235
22:20—The Wait Is Over! 235

Complete Song List

Meditation	Song Title	Link
You Are Forgiven	"Forgiveness"	https://youtu.be/olbCpyOCQEo
God Rules Everything	"O Worship the King"	https://youtu.be/We9aR22C9Bl
Don't Panic — He's Got You!	"Refuge"	https://vimeo.com/232853172
How to Pray	"My Help, My God"	https://sandramccracken.bandcamp.com/track/my-help-my-god-psalm-42
Knowledge that Will Change Your World	"He Is God"	https://www.reverbnation.com/susancalderazzo/songs
Live by Every Word	"The Word Is So Near"	https://youtu.be/biXrKOalJq4
Your Troubled Heart	"Sweet Comfort"	https://sandramccracken.bandcamp.com/track/sweet-comfort
Sharing the Story	"Add to the Beauty"	https://youtu.be/9htYsEblADU
Prayer Requests	"Come People of the Risen King"	https://store.gettymusic.com/us/song/come-people-of-the-risen-king/
Looking for a Better Place	"I Can Only Imagine"	https://youtu.be/Rlu-a1lgeTo
Our Ultimate Question	"Though You Slay Me"	https://youtu.be/qyUPz6_TciY

Meditation	Song Title	Link
God's Answer	"The Job Suite"	https://youtu.be/OuqOx3B4WYO
I Know Whom I Have Believed	"I Know Whom I Have Believed"	https://youtu.be/_bRV3J4n8cc
'Tis So Sweet to Trust in Jesus	"'Tis So Sweet to Trust in Jesus"	https://youtu.be/ZiEqKpN9OW4
Your Helper is Here!	"Come, O Come Thou Holy Spirit"	https://youtu.be/p-jJqhz1bgg
Unfulfilled	"Our Hope Endures"	https://youtu.be/n1mu3FOdQzO
All Will Be Well	"All Must Be Well"	https://youtu.be/Y5OEDNEJvTA
Never Give Up	"Everlasting God"	https://youtu.be/QVmaLtyOSao
My Peace I Give	"It Is Well with My Soul"	https://youtu.be/GTa3p3DiEag
The Peace of God	"Perfect Peace"	https://youtu.be/UF2iilrWBbl
When You Are Weak	"The Weight of the World"	https://youtu.be/mvTZpYTUNtl
Searching for Signs of Redemption	"There You Are"	https://youtu.be/lVHCWW-aCNs
When God Said No	"Thy Will Be Done"	https://indeliblegrace.bandcamp.com/track/thy-will-be-done
Steadfast	"Steadfast"	https://youtu.be/SlsFC6RzUNk
The Embrace of the Father	"The Communion Hymn"	https://youtu.be/S1rQy1TrgXl
Jesus Wept	"Come to Jesus"	https://youtu.be/ZyaA_ttbl8E
Worth Waiting For	"It's Hard to Wait"	https://youtu.be/HbMsm328cu8
The Gentleness of Jesus	"He Leadeth Me"	https://youtu.be/Zwm7MlUtDaO

Meditation	Song Title	Link
Mat-Friends	"What a Friend We Have in Jesus"	https://youtu.be/znWu2HCJ92c
Termites, Tumors, and Other Hidden Dangers	"Mighty to Save"	https://youtu.be/W1jmqVU4RDo
Count Your Losses	"We Will Feast in the House of Zion"	https://youtu.be/ujVBV3lNSbQ
Count Your Blessings	"Blessings"	https://youtu.be/JKPeoPiK9XE
Return to Normal	"All Things New"	https://youtu.be/FhpQN9JXNXA
A Good Scar Story	"When I Survey the Wondrous Cross"	https://youtu.be/xLXx2CJ_drs
Everyday Miracles	"How Great Is Our God"	https://youtu.be/DpIcqoKOz2M
Tough Decisions	"The Perfect Wisdom of our God"	https://youtu.be/hSnzYnOe6kI
The First Enemy: Satan	"A Mighty Fortress Is Our God"	https://youtu.be/bONV_YZCKdg
The Final Enemy: Death	"Death Be Not Proud"	https://youtu.be/9ID7dmCiAgw
The Wait Is Over	"Great Rejoicing"	https://rainforroots.bandcamp.com/track/great-rejoicing.

ENJOYED THIS BOOK? Reading a borrowed copy, or want to gift a friend? Please consider these ways to let others know:

Purchase your own copy at favorite booksellers, or visit www.elizabethturnage.com/TheWaitingRoom

CONSIDER SHARING THIS BOOK WITH OTHERS:

Share or mention on your social media platforms. Use the hashtag #TheWaitingRoomdevotional .

Write a book review on Amazon or Goodreads.

Share this message on Facebook, Twitter or Instagram: "I loved #TheWaitingRoomDevotional by Elizabeth Reynolds Turnage #etstory.

WANT MORE GOOD GOSPEL-CENTERED RESOURCES?

Get free planners, story starters, prayer cards, and more. Sign up at http://eepurl.com/b__teX

Other books by
Elizabeth Reynolds Turnage

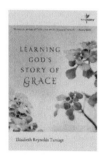 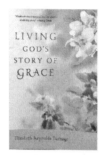 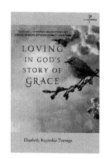

Learning in God's Story of Grace: P & R, 2010
Living in God's Story of Grace: P & R, 2011
Loving in God's Story of Grace: P & R, 2014.